ACSM'S EXEI
IS MEDICINE™:
A Clinician's Guide to Exercise Prescription

EDITED B

Steven J

Professor, Dep
School of Med

Edward

Director, Outp
Assistant Prof
Harvard Medi
Assistant Phys
Adjunct Scient
Jean Mayer U
Tufts Universi
Founder and

	DATE		

The Institu

Publishe
www.insti

org

RICAN COLLEGE
PORTS MEDICINE
w.acsm.org

Supporte
www.apo

vw.acsm.org

ms & Wilkins

BAKER & TAYLOR

Acquisitions Editor: Sonya Seigafuse
Managing Editor: Kerry Barrett
Project Manager: Alicia Jackson
Senior Manufacturing Manager: Benjamin Rivera
Marketing Manager: Kimberly Schonberger
Designer: Terry Mallon
Cover Designer: Scott Rattray
Production Service: Circle Graphics

ACSM's Publications Committee Chair: Jeffrey L. Roitman, Ed.D., FACSM
ACSM's Group Publisher: Kerry O'Rourke

Printed in the U.S.A.

978-1-58255-739-7
1-58255-739-X
Library of Congress Cataloging-in-Publication Data
available upon request

*Care has been taken to confirm the accuracy of the information presented and to describe generally
accepted practices. However, the authors, editors, and publisher are not responsible for errors or
omissions or for any consequences from application of the information in this book and make no
warranty, expressed or implied, with respect to the currency, completeness, or accuracy of the con-
tents of the publication. Application of the information in a particular situation remains the professional responsibility of the practitioner.*

*The authors, editors, and publisher have exerted every effort to ensure that drug selection and
dosage set forth in this text are in accordance with current recommendations and practice at the
time of publication. However, in view of ongoing research, changes in government regulations, and
the constant flow of information relating to drug therapy and drug reactions, the reader is urged to
check the package insert for each drug for any change in indications and dosage and for added
warnings and precautions. This is particularly important when the recommended agent is a new or
infrequently employed drug.*

*Some drugs and medical devices presented in the publication have Food and Drug Administration
(FDA) clearance for limited use in restricted research settings. It is the responsibility of health care
providers to ascertain the FDA status of each drug or device planned for use in their clinical practice.*

To purchase additional copies of this book, call our customer service department at **(800)
638-3030** or fax orders to **(301) 223-2320.** International customers should call **(301) 223-2300.**

Visit Lippincott Williams & Wilkins on the Internet: at LWW.com. Lippincott Williams &
Wilkins customer service representatives are available from 8:30 am to 6 pm, EST.

10 9 8 7 6 5 4 3

RRS0911

DEDICATION

For Chezna, and all of the other regular exercisers, past, present
and future, for whom this book has been written.

S.J.

To Alison,
My exercise partner and personal prescription
for health, love, and happiness.

E.P.

CONTRIBUTORS

Jennifer Capell, PT, MSc, MPH
Institute of Lifestyle Medicine
Boston, Massachusetts

Steven Jonas, MD, MPH, MS, FNYAS
Professor of Preventive Medicine and
*   the Graduate Program in Public Health*
School of Medicine
Stony Brook University
Stony Brook, New York

Evonne Kaplan-Liss, MD, MPH, FAAP
Director, Pediatric Environmental Center of
*   Clinical Excellence at Stony Brook*
Research Assistant Professor in the Graduate
*   Program in Public Health, Preventive*
*   Medicine, Pediatrics, and Journalism*
School of Medicine
State University of New York at Stony Brook
Stony Brook, New York

Edward M. Phillips, MD
Director, Outpatient Medical Services
Spaulding Rehabilitation Hospital Network
Boston, Massachusetts
Assistant Professor
Department of Physical Medicine and
*   Rehabilitation*
Harvard Medical School
Assistant Physiatrist
Massachusetts General Hospital
Adjunct Scientist
Jean Mayer USDA Human Nutrition Research
*   Center on Aging*
Tufts University
Boston, Massachusetts

Mary Ellen Renna, MD, FAAP
Physician Nutrition Specialist
Woodbury, New York

The following organizations have endorsed this project:

- Institute of Lifestyle Medicine, Harvard Medical School
- American College of Preventive Medicine
- Kaiser Permanente
- Apollo Hospitals Group
- American Alliance for Health, Physical Education, Recreation and Dance
- American Council on Exercise
- American Physical Therapy Association
- IDEA Health & Fitness Association
- Medical Fitness Association
- National Association for Health and Fitness
- National Athletic Trainers' Association
- National Coalition for Promoting Physical Activity
- National Strength and Conditioning Association

The following organization supports this project:

- President's Council on Physical Fitness and Sports

CONTENTS

FOREWORD

Exercise is Medicine™: A Clinician's Guide to Exercise Prescription

By Robert E. Sallis, MD, FACSM

"Eating alone will not keep a man well; he must also take exercise. For food and exercise . . . work together to produce health." Wise words. I was reminded that this prescription is credited not to the American College of Sports Medicine (ACSM), or the American Medical Association (AMA), or numerous other stakeholders who advance health daily for mankind. As ACSM's Historian, Jack W. Berryman, PhD, FACSM, so pointedly noted, it was none other than Hippocrates who gave this advice in his book *Regimen* in 400 B.C.E.

Today, ACSM, the AMA and many other supporting organizations are calling on all physicians and healthcare workers to make physical activity and exercise a standard part of a disease prevention and treatment medical paradigm in the United States . . . and the world.

As a nation, we have a lot at stake in getting our citizens to take the "Exercise Pill." The cost of inactivity is staggering, with an estimated 250,000 premature deaths annually in the U.S. directly attributed to inactivity and the costs of medical care for inactive patients dwarfing that required to care for active ones. Further, we are looking at a generation of children who are much less fit than their parents and with the potential to be the first not to live longer than their parents. I believe that physical inactivity will become the greatest public health problem of our time if we do not take action.

This book is an important educational tool for physicians and other clinical healthcare professionals committed to advancing the principles of the Exercise is Medicine™ initiative. This book will help guide doctors to prescribe exercise to their patients. A recent survey conducted of the public by ACSM found that nearly two-thirds of patients (65%) would be more interested in exercising to stay healthy if advised by their doctor and given additional resources. However, only four out of ten physicians (41%) talk to their patients about the importance of exercise, but don't always offer suggestions on the best ways to be physically active.

The time has come for physicians to become strong advocates for exercise. They must ask about it at every patient visit and a patient's activity level should be looked at as a vital sign, because it is one of the best indicators of a person's health and longevity. Patients should be advised to engage in the ACSM's recommended 30 minutes of moderate exercise (such as a brisk walk) on most (five or more) days each week. This is especially important in patients who have, or are risk for, chronic diseases like diabetes or heart disease. This message should be the same, regardless of medical provider or specialty and this concept should be embraced and reinforced throughout all of organized medicine.

On behalf of the American College of Sports Medicine, I want to thank the American Medical Association for joining ACSM in making this program an important joint effort. I also want to thank this book's authors—Steven Jonas, MD, MPH, MS, FNYAS, and Edward M. Phillips, MD—for dedicating their time and talents to produce this book. I thank Evonne Kaplan-Liss MD, MPH, FAAP, and Mary Ellen Renna, MD, FAAP, for lending their expertise in authoring the chapter on pediatric exercise. And, as no successful project is so without much support, ACSM duly recognizes the organizations that cooperatively present this work: Harvard Medical School's Institute of Lifestyle Medicine and the American College of Preventive Medicine. You can also find an impressive and extensive list of supporting organizations and companies on page v.

I hope this book will encourage you to prescribe exercise to all of your patients!

Sincerely

Robert Sallis, MD, FACSM
President, American College of Sports Medicine
2007–2008

PREFACE

Welcome to Exercise is Medicine™. In 2007 the original "Exercise is Medicine™ Task Force" set forth the Vision of the enterprise as follows (1):

"To make physical activity and exercise a standard part of a disease prevention and treatment medical paradigm in the United States.

"For physical activity to be considered by all healthcare providers as a vital sign in every patient visit, and that patients are effectively counseled and referred as to their physical activity and health needs, thus leading to overall improvement in the public's health and long-term reduction in healthcare cost.

"Exercise is Medicine™ will be a sustainable national initiative that:

1. Creates broad awareness that exercise is indeed medicine.
2. Makes 'level of physical activity' a standard vital sign question in each patient visit.
3. Helps physicians and other healthcare providers to become consistently effective in counseling and referring patients as to their physical activity needs.
4. Leads to policy changes in public and private sectors that support physical activity counseling and referrals in clinical settings.
5. Produces an expectation among the public and patients that their healthcare providers should and will ask about and prescribe exercise.
6. Appropriately encourages physicians and other healthcare providers to be physically active themselves.

"The Program Elements as originally laid out were:

Area 1. Make available tools, training, and referral mechanisms for physicians and other healthcare providers.
Area 2. Strengthen the science and evidence for the efficacy of exercise prescription in healthcare settings.
Area 3. Pursue policy interventions that support Exercise is Medicine™.
Area 4. Stage patient advocacy and marketing campaigns
Area 5. Build coalitions and partnerships.
Area 6. Identify, develop, and disseminate "what works" models for patients as well as entire communities.
Area 7. Create a Web site with strategy, content, and functions that support all the program elements of Exercise is Medicine™"

This book is designed specifically to assist physicians and indeed all healthcare professionals who are interested in helping patients and clients to become regular exercisers in learning how they can most effectively do that. Our book covers the regular exercise waterfront, from helping you to organize your own mind-set for the process, to mobilizing patient/client motivation, which we see as the key element in the whole enterprise, through the nuts and bolts of what to do and how to do it, finishing up with how to have fun as a regular exerciser. We go in depth into both the *lifestyle exercise* approach to exercising regularly and the *structured exercise* approach.

Several technical notes. First, there is repetition in this book. It is intentional. Most readers of this type of book don't read it from cover to cover, and we would like to increase the chances that each of you will have the chance to learn and reflect upon its most important points, analyses, and recommendations. Let us repeat that: there is repetition throughout this book. Second, we understand that some readers refer to the people they take care of as their "patients," others as their "clients." To avoid clumsiness, we use the single term "patients" to refer to both. Finally, we know that many readers have a very limited amount of time to devote to this subject in the course of their clinical practices. Therefore we have organized a set of "Three-Minute Drills" and similar materials under other headings that appear throughout the book. They cover the theory in "three-minute" or similar chunks of time, what your patients can think about in three minutes or so that will help them, and what you can do on the practical side with your patients in three minutes or so. As we said at the outset, welcome to the world of Exercise is Medicine™.

ACKNOWLEDGMENTS

We would like to thank, first and foremost, the American College of Sports Medicine and its leadership, most especially Robert Sallis, MD, Past President, who initiated this project and James Whitehead, Executive Vice President, for the confidence they placed in us in asking us to be the authors for this book. Many thanks to D. Mark Robertson, former Assistant Executive Vice President–*Publishing, Editorial Services, Membership & Chapter Services, ACSM,* for both his excellent guidance and encouragement throughout the writing process. We would like to thank Ralph Bovard, MD, MPH, and his ACSM review panel for the insight and excellent suggestions they had for us in their review of the original manuscript. Their work made the book that much stronger. Walter Thompson, MD, provided us with the benefit of his expertise at a number of stages along the way; thus special thanks to him also. To our editors at Lippincott Williams & Wilkins, principally Sonya Seigafuse and Kerry Barrett, many thanks for their consistently high quality work in bringing our book into being and managing its production. We would also like to thank the copy-editing staff, lead by Joanne Revak, for a fine job at that stage of the book's development. Our gratitude is extended to the Harvard Medical School Department of Physical Medicine and Rehabilitation for providing a grant to support our energetic and very capable research assistant Jennifer Capell, PT, MSc, MPH, and to Mary Alice Hanford in the Department's Institute of Lifestyle Medicine for her valuable editing and input at a number of points along the way. Finally, we would like to thank the late Ronald Davis, MD, President of the American Medical Association during the time when we got this book off the ground, for his support and encouragement for the project.

Steven Jonas MD, MPH, MS, FNYAS,
and **Edward Phillips, MD**
November 18, 2008

Reference

1. Exercise is Medicine™ Task Force, "About Exercise Is Medicine™," http://www.exerciseismedicine.org/about.htm (Feb., 2008).

Introduction: What This Book Is About

Steven Jonas

LET'S GET GOING!

This book is about change and how to make it, choices to be made and how to make them, new vistas for life and how to embrace them, all in the realm of regular physical activity. In this realm, on both the health professional and the patient[1] sides, one size does NOT fit all. The book is about making changes in the way you think and act in dealing with your patients on the subject of regular exercise, and the choices you have in doing so. It's about the changes that your patients can and will make to help themselves become regular exercisers, and the choices they have in doing so. It's about how you can best assist them in going about making those changes and choices.

Of the choices to be made, all are of the type that we like to call "a choice of goods." We present a set of change-making/choice-making tools for both you and your patients to use, to make the changes that will suit both you and your patients best. There are many options available that will lead both you and your patients to a healthy result. We will help you and, through you, your patients, to identify them. One of our favorite sayings in this realm is: "The best exercise for **you** is the exercise that is **best** for you."

ADVICE: WHAT WORKS AND WHAT DOESN'T

The American media are filled with advice about *how to* make personal health-promoting behavior changes. You see it every day, both health-specific and general, at the supermarket checkout counter, on TV, on the Web, and in countless magazines. There are tons of advice on: *how to* exercise: choice of activities and sports, schedules, techniques, and equipment; *how to* lose weight: diets, food choices, and advice on shopping, cooking, and *how to* eat;

---

[1]As also noted in the Preface, different health professionals use different terms in referring to those whom they serve. For simplicity's sake, throughout this book we use the term "patient" to signify all of them.

how to quit smoking, and so on. There is also a great deal of information available on the consequences of unhealthy lifestyles. Yet, Americans continue to engage frequently in unhealthy behaviors leading to those unhealthy lifestyles, and the rates of doing so are increasing. Thus, at all ages, as is very well-known, at an alarming rate we are becoming a heavier and a significantly less-active population. This is a change in the profile of the population that is already having a significant negative economic as well as negative health impact. Unless we make some serious attempts to reverse it, it will only get more serious over time. It has thus become apparent that if most people are to achieve success in making health-promoting lifestyle and behavior changes, simply providing advice on techniques, schedules, and diets—that is on the "how to's" and on "what-is-good-for-you-and-what-is-not," is simply not sufficient. If it were, we as a nation would not be where we are in the realm of physical activity and fitness, nor in overweight and obesity. Thus it is that relatively few people are regular exercisers despite the mountains of available exercise information focused on "exercise is good for you" and the specifics of "what to do" in terms of activities and sports.

Why is that so? The answer is straightforward. Before a person can get started on any program—for regular exercise, for weight loss, for what have you—they need to get themselves *motivated* to do it. *Mobilizing motivation* is a multistep process, one with which we deal at length in this book. Mastering it is central to achieving success. However, as experience shows, it is the hardest part of getting going and keeping on going. The motivation mobilization process is more than just wishing something. It involves, for starters, self-assessment, realistically defining success for oneself, and undertaking, as its central element, goal-setting.

We spend the better part of four chapters in this book going into the subject of motivation in detail. Virtually none of the information generally available elsewhere deals with it in any detail at all. Is it any wonder then that most of that oh-so-widely available information goes to waste?

THE ROLE OF THE CLINICIAN

The matter of mobilizing motivation is where you, the clinician, have a central role. It is difficult for the average person to learn about the health-promoting motivational process just from reading. For example, most people do not learn on their own about the centrality of careful goal-setting in personal health promotion. (If they could, we would not have nearly as many unsuccessful weight-losers and "I-tried-it-but-it-didn't-work" non-exercisers as we have.) Some can do it on their own, but many more will be successful if they can participate in the process of guided discovery that you can provide for them. Even just mentioning regular exercise in the course of a patient visit can have a very helpful effect in helping that patient to get going. This book is designed to help you become an effective promoter of regular exercise for your patients in the course of your regular practice and to help you to effectively provide the exercise prescription for your patients, *within the limits of time that every busy practitioner faces.*

There is a range of roles that you can play in this regard. Three of the principal roles you as clinician can adopt in helping your patients to become regular exercisers are "The Three Ms: Mentioning, Motivating, Modeling." Simply mentioning regular exercise on a regular basis with a referral to outside resources is for some patients all they need. Providing some more detailed help on the motivational process and how to mobilize it, is, as noted, very important for many patients. Then, if you have the time and interest to do so, you can get into the details of choice of activities and sports, schedules, and equipment. Beyond that, if you are not one already, you can, and perhaps should, decide to become a role model, too, if you have the time and interest for that as well.

You may simply decide to use the several paper forms for the exercise prescription that we provide for you. You may decide, on occasion with selected patients, to spend a bit more than the time it takes simply to hand them an exercise prescription. Or you may go further and decide to undertake some significant changes in the way you conduct your practice and organize it, too. We will help you to learn how to do all of these elements effectively. Just as your patients will decide what they want to do and how far they will go with exercising regularly, so too will you make the choices about just what you want to do in the course of your practice to help them.

There are a variety of different forms of activities and sports that patients can use for exercising regularly. There are important details for all of them that can be useful for you to know, again depending upon how much time you have to devote to the effort. Some patients will be most comfortable with the "lifestyle exercise" approach, in which they incorporate short bouts of regular exercise, like using the stairs instead of the elevator and parking the car at the far end of the parking lot, into their everyday activities. Others will engage in leisure-time, scheduled, regular exercise using a sport or other athletic activity in "The Scheduled Training Exercise Program" (TSTEP) approach. Understanding that **the hard part of regular exercise is the *regular,* not the *exercise,*** is essential if you are going to be effective for your patients. We will guide you through all of the details as well as presenting our overall philosophy.

WHY THE PRESCRIPTION

Considering the thousands of articles documenting the benefits of exercise for physiologic, metabolic, and psychological health, if exercise were a pill everyone should take it. Indeed, *Exercise **is** Medicine.* As such, in this book we hold that all clinicians (not just licensed physicians) should prescribe this vital "medication" to every patient as needed, at every visit, and as appropriate. As we discuss the serious side effects of inactivity, we argue that the impetus to prescribe exercise is equivalent to the need to prescribe a lifesaving treatment to a dying patient. It is no longer acceptable for clinicians to be mute on this subject.

For physicians, the prescription pad is a familiar and comfortable way of transmitting authority and the import of a recommendation—whether it is for a medication or a referral to another professional such as a therapist to obtain a specific treatment. Similarly, the exercise prescription directs patients to initiate, maintain, or increase their level of physical activity. As we detail in the book, the structure of this prescription mimics that of medication prescriptions. All clinicians are led through a means to effectively and efficiently prescribe exercise that is acceptable to patients and safe for them to pursue.

A QUICK TOUR OF THE BOOK

In this book we first discuss the central elements of clinician engagement and counseling. We show you, too, (in Chapters 1 and 2) how to reorganize your practice, should you wish to, to further and more intensively facilitate the regular provision of the exercise prescription in it—although such reorganization is certainly not essential for providing much needed and very useful advice and counsel on regular exercise for your patients. In this regard, given the wide variety of clinical practitioners dealing with this subject, for clinicians who have widely differing amounts of available time, interest, and principal foci of their practices, it will be *different strokes for different folks*.

We then move on to the broad agenda of bringing your patients through a three-stage progression (Figure 1): first, in the Foundation Phase by ensuring the safety of patients initiating or increasing physical activity (Chapter 3) and, second, to Mobilizing Motivation (Chapters 4, 5, and 6). In fact, we present two approaches to the latter subject, in both of which we have confidence. You can choose one or the other, or create some combination of both that works for you as well as for your patients.

We then move on to the Becoming Active Phase, with details of scheduling and exercise/sports programming for both the "lifestyle" and "scheduled leisure-time" approaches, starting from inactivity on to reaching the ACSM/AHA/HHS minimum goals of physical activity (see p. 5 and Chapters 7 and 8). In the final phase, Staying Active Phase, we help you guide your patients from the ACSM/AHA/HHS minimum levels of activity (Chapter 9). In keeping with the theme of choices, we present in Chapter 10 a more structured exercise prescription to assist your patients across the spectrum from sedentary to habitual vigorous exercise. In Chapters 11 and 12, choosing activities,

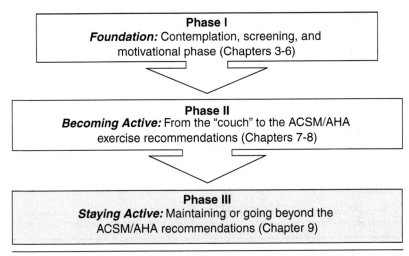

Figure 1 • Lifestyle Changes: From Sedentary to Active

sports, techniques, and equipment are Chapter 13 covers the considerations in providing the exercise prescription in disease treatment and management and in special conditions such as pregnancy and old age. Chapter 14 considers the special needs of children, in particular how to make regular exercise a family affair. We finish off in Chapter 15 with how to make regular exercise fun.

As noted, from time to time we will present you with a "three-minute drill" that will be either a summary of major thoughts/constructs in the book that you can go over in your head in three minutes (or less), or a formulation that you can use with patients in the course of preparing the Exercise Prescription with and for them, in the course of three minutes (or less). You will find the first two of these in Three-Minute Drills Introduction-1 and Introduction-2.

THREE-MINUTE DRILL, INTRODUCTION – 1

When a Patient Asks, "Why Exercise?"

1. It makes you feel better.
2. It makes you look better.
3. It makes you feel better about yourself.
4. It reduces your risk of getting a variety of diseases and negative health conditions, such as heart disease, diabetes, certain forms of cancer, obesity, high blood pressure, and osteoporosis.
5. It helps in the amelioration and management of a similar list of diseases and negative health conditions.

THREE-MINUTE DRILL, INTRODUCTION – 2

Regular Exercise: 7 Major Benefits

1. *Regular* Exercise is the only way to "get in shape."
2. *Regular* Exercise is essential for managing your weight in a healthy manner.
3. *Regular* Exercise can help you to feel younger and act that way too.
4. *Regular* Exercise strengthens your muscles and builds physical endurance.
5. *Regular* Exercise can help you to sleep better.
6. *Regular* Exercise can help spark your sex life.
7. *Regular* Exercise can be fun, if you let it be fun!

For an overview supporting both Three-Minute Drills, and providing much more useful information, see http://www.nlm.nih.gov/medlineplus/exerciseandphysicalfitness.html

EXERCISE AND HEALTH

We do not present the extensive data on the positive relationship between regular exercise and health in any detail in this book. In June 2008, in preparation for the development of the U.S. Department of Health and Human Services (USDHHS) "Physical Activity Guidelines for Americans" that were released in the fall of 2008, the Office of Disease Prevention and Health Promotion of the USDHHS published the most comprehensive review ever carried out of the epidemiological, medical, and social science of regular exercise and its role in promoting human health (1). Over 8000 articles reporting the benefits of exercise were reviewed in preparing this report.

In summary, moderate physical activity can substantially reduce the risk of developing or dying from heart disease, diabetes, several forms of cancer, and high blood pressure (2, 3, 4, 5). It is important in the prevention and management of overweight/obesity and osteoporosis. The improvement in mobility that accompanies it is important in maintaining functional independence for healthy aging, as well as for protecting against lower back pain. It also reduces falls among older adults; helps to relieve the pain of arthritis; reduces symptoms of anxiety and depression; and is associated with fewer hospitalizations, physician visits, and medications. On average, physically active people outlive those who are inactive. As the ACSM has said (6): "Physical activity offers one of the greatest opportunities for people to extend years of active independent life and reduces functional limitations. . . . A substantial body of scientific evidence indicates that regular physical activity can bring dramatic health benefits to people of all ages and abilities, with these benefits extending over the life span . . . and improve the quality of life."

For a summary of the reasons for engaging in regular exercise, see Three-Minute Drills Intro.-1 and Intro.-2. Of these reasons, perhaps the most important is not about bringing risk factors under control or "getting in shape" for the sake of being in shape. Rather, it is what regular exercise does for the mind: it makes one feel better and feel better about oneself. An important aspect of that is that, for many, it makes one look better too.

HOW MUCH, TO GET STARTED

For some years now, the American College of Sports Medicine and the American Heart Association have jointly published recommendations for the minimum weekly levels of regular exercise that promote health. A summary of these recommendations, as of mid-year 2008, is found in Table 1. Throughout this book we refer to these recommendations as our baselines. In the fall of 2008, the United States Department of Health and Human Services released the first federal recommendations for physical activity (Table 2). The findings of the HHS closely follow the ACSM/AHA guidelines. The minor variations in the amount of daily activity and their recommendations relative to specific groups, including older adults and children, will allow you to further tailor your exercise prescription to your patient.

BEING A REGULAR EXERCISER

Being a regular exerciser is like being on a never-ending journey. Many miles are covered, many hours are spent, and many new vistas are uncovered, in both the mind and the world outside. But no final destination is ever reached, because for the regular exerciser, by definition there cannot ever be one. If you, the healthcare professional reading this book, are a regular exerciser yourself, you already know about the never-ending journey. But whether or not you are yet on the journey of regular exercise for yourself, by deciding to read this book you have begun a parallel journey into a world that is new for many healthcare practitioners—one in which exercise promotion is a significant part of one's practice. To that world, we say "welcome!" And having been regular exercisers ourselves, as have been so many members of the American College of Sports Medicine, we heartily recommend that, if you are not presently a regular exerciser yourself, you seriously consider becoming one, both for your own benefit and that of your patients.

Thus this book addresses two different kinds of experiences: yours and your patients'. For both clinician and patient, this book provides a series of easy-to-do, easy-to-use programs for exercising regularly (again, see Chapters 7–10). Beyond this, hopefully the book will also help you to organize your own thoughts about regular exercise; develop a system, from simple to more complex, for introducing and using its promotion as part of your regular practice;

TABLE 1   American College of Sports Medicine and American Heart Association Guidelines for Regular Exercise; Health Promoting Minimums

Guidelines for Healthy Adults Under Age 65; Basic Recommendations from ACSM and AHA:

Do moderately intense cardio 30 minutes a day, five days a week

Or

Do vigorously intense cardio 20 minutes a day, 3 days a week

And

Do eight to 10 strength-training exercises, eight to 12 repetitions of each exercise twice a week.

- Because of the dose-response relation between physical activity and health, persons who wish to further improve their personal fitness, reduce their risk for chronic diseases and disabilities, or prevent unhealthy weight gain will likely benefit by exceeding the minimum recommended amount of physical activity.

Physical activity above the recommended minimum amount provides even greater health benefits.

Moderate-intensity physical activity means working hard enough to raise your heart rate and break a sweat, yet still being able to carry on a conversation. It should be noted that to lose weight or maintain weight loss, 60 to 90 minutes of physical activity may be necessary. The 30-minute recommendation is for the average healthy adult to maintain health and reduce the risk for chronic disease.

Guidelines for Adults Over Age 65 (or Adults 50–64 With Chronic Conditions, Such as Arthritis); Basic Recommendations from ACSM and AHA:

Do moderately intense aerobic exercise 30 minutes a day, five days a week

Or

Do vigorously intense aerobic exercise 20 minutes a day, 3 days a week

And

Do eight to 10 strength-training exercises, 10–15 repetitions of each exercise twice to three times per week

And

If you are at risk of falling, perform balance exercises

And

Have a physical activity plan.

- Because of the dose-response relation between physical activity and health, persons who wish to further improve their personal fitness, reduce their risk for chronic diseases and disabilities, or prevent unhealthy weight gain will likely benefit by exceeding the minimum recommended amount of physical activity.

TABLE 1 *(Continued)*

- Physical activity above the recommended minimum amount provides even greater health benefits.

Both aerobic and muscle-strengthening activity is critical for healthy aging. **Moderate-intensity aerobic exercise** means working hard at about a level-six intensity on a scale of 10. You should still be able to carry on a conversation during exercise.

Older adults or adults with chronic conditions should develop an **activity plan** with a health professional to manage risks and take therapeutic needs into account. This will maximize the benefits of physical activity and ensure your safety.

Starting an Exercise Program

Starting an exercise program can sound like a daunting task, but just remember that your main goal is to meet the basic physical activity recommendations: 30 minutes of moderate-intensity physical activity at least five days per week, or vigorous-intensity activity at least three days per week, and strength training two to three times per week. Choose activities that appeal to you and will make exercise fun. **Walking** is a great, easy way to do moderate-intensity physical activity.

Source: These guidelines, and additional detail/commentary on them, can be found at http://www.acsm.org/, "Physical Activity Guidelines from ACSM and AHA."

and deal with the central problem of motivation, for your patients and, if needed, for yourself as well. If you happen not to be a regular exerciser yourself now, you can certainly use the nuts and bolts part of this book as your personal guide to becoming one.

SOME DEFINITIONS

Physical activity is "any body movement produced by skeletal muscles that results in a substantive increase over the resting energy expenditure." *Leisure-time physical activity* is "an activity undertaken in the individual's discretionary time that leads to any substantial increase in the total daily energy expenditure." *Scheduled exercise* is "a form of leisure-time physical activity that is usually performed on a repeated basis over an extended period of time (exercise training) with a specific external objective such as the improvement of fitness, physical performance, or health" (2). *Fitness* is the ability to do physical work over time, using the musculoskeletal and cardiovascular systems.

TABLE 2 U.S. Department of Health and Human Services Physical Activity Guidelines for Americans 2008

The HHS recommends that in order to promote and maintain health, all healthy adults ages 18–65 years need:

- Moderate-intensity aerobic activity for a minimum of 30 min on five days each week
- Or vigorous-intensity aerobic activity for a minimum of 20 min on three days each week
- Or a combination of moderate- and vigorous-intensity activity . . . to meet this recommendation.
- Because of the dose–response relation between physical activity and health, persons who wish to further improve their personal fitness, reduce their risk for chronic diseases and disabilities, or prevent unhealthy weight gain will likely benefit by exceeding the minimum recommended amount of physical activity.
- Physical activity above the recommended minimum amount provides even greater health benefits.

Source: United States Department of Health and Human Services, October 2008. "Physical Activity Guidelines for Americans."

Regular exercise can also be engaged in as part of daily living, with various activities like brisk walking and stair-climbing built into one's regular routine. As noted above, this is known as *lifestyle* exercise. Noting these distinctions, we shall use the terms *physical activity* and *exercise* interchangeably throughout the book. It is important to note as well that *regularity*, exercising on a repeated basis over an extended period of time, is included in the standard definition for exercise. *Sessions* (particularly of the lifestyle exercise type of regular exercise), *workouts*, and *going to the gym* are terms that are used interchangeably with regular exercise throughout this book.

Exercise is considered *aerobic* when it is intense enough to lead to a significant increase in muscle oxygen uptake. Exercise done at a level of intensity below aerobic is any physical activity above the normal resting state that involves one or more major muscle groups, is sustained, but not so intense as to cause a significant increase in muscle oxygen uptake. *Anaerobic* exercise is intense physical activity, necessarily of very short duration (usually measured in seconds), fueled by energy sources solely within the contracting muscles, and does not depend upon the use of inhaled oxygen as an energy source. For the most part, other than for lifters of heavy weights and certain competitive athletes such as short-distance swimmers and track sprinters, anaerobic exercise is not a factor in regular, health-promoting exercise. However, it should be noted that the more intense the activity, that is the more aerobic it is, the more benefit there is to be gained from it, particularly as one ages (7).

THE RISKS OF REGULAR EXERCISE IN THE OTHERWISE HEALTHY PATIENT

Along with its many benefits, regular exercise carries with it a few risks as well. However, virtually all of them are preventable or at least modifiable. Injury is the most common risk, of which there are two types, extrinsic and intrinsic. Extrinsic injury is that caused by an external factor, *e.g.,* a car hitting a cyclist. Intrinsic injury is that caused by the nature of the sport or activity, *e.g.,* a stress fracture is incurred while running. The former type of injury can be modified or prevented by taking certain safety precautions, primarily of the commonsense variety, such as never wearing a headset when riding a bicycle (so that one can hear cars coming) and always wearing a helmet (so that if one's head bounces in a fall, the chances of serious injury to it are significantly reduced). The latter type can be prevented or at least mitigated by the use of proper equipment (for example, in running, wearing shoes properly designed, correctly fitted, and not over-worn, and maintaining moderation in distance, intensity, and speed). The most common cause of injury in most of the activities and sports used for regular exercise, such as running, fast walking, cycling, and swimming is overuse—trying to go too far, too fast, too frequently. The risk of such injuries can be very significantly lowered by choosing a suitable sport and a workout schedule.

There is also, of course, the risk of aggravating an underlying pathological condition that is not yet clinically apparent, such as coronary artery disease. As discussed in detail in Chapters 3 and 13, such risks can be mitigated by a) appropriate screening for patients with risk factors for preclinical pathological conditions, and b) making sure that patients are aware of "when to stop," "when is too much indeed too much," and when to seek medical attention.

BALANCE AND EXERCISE

An important key to success in regularly exercising **over time** is found in one word: balance. If a person does not exercise or does not exercise enough, she will not get its benefits. If she exercises too much, or does a kind of exercise that is not right for her or that does not fit into her body's balanced scheme of things and the balance of her life, exercise can be harmful. If exercise is to be beneficial, health-promoting, and to contributive to our feelings of well-being, it must be balanced in two ways. First, the exercise(s) and/or activities that we choose to do must be the right one(s) for us, our bodies, our minds, our schedules, and the other things that are going on in our lives. Second, both the amount and intensity of the exercise(s) that we choose to do must fall within the limits of what is healthy for *us*. Doing this will help us to achieve balance.

CONCLUSION

Let us leave the last words of this chapter to one of the greatest minds of the 18th century, if not of all time. It did not require modern medical science to lead Thomas Jefferson to come to the following conclusion about both the value of health and the relationship of regular exercise to it. He said (8):

> Without health, there is no happiness. And attention to health, then, should take the place of every other object. The time necessary to secure this by active exercises should be devoted to it in preference to every other pursuit. I know the difficulty with which a strenuous man tears himself from his studies at any given moment of the day; but his happiness, and that of his family depend on it. The most uninformed mind, with a healthy body is happier than the wisest valetudinarian" [that is a "sickly or weak person, esp. one who is constantly and morbidly concerned with his health" (9)].

References

1. Physical Activity Guidelines Advisory Committee (US). Physical Activity Guidelines Advisory Committee report, 2008 [Internet]. Washington: US Department of Health and Human Services; 2008 Jun [cited 2008 Sep 22]. 683 p. Available from: http://www.health.gov/paguidelines/Report/pdf/CommitteeReport.pdf
2. Bouchard C, Shephard RJ, Stephens T, ed. Physical activity, fitness, and health: international proceedings and consensus statement. Champaign (IL): Human Kinetics Publishers; 1994. 1055 p.
3. Project PACE. Physical activity. San Diego (CA): San Diego State University Foundation and San Diego Center for Health Interventions; 1999
4. Centers for Disease Control and Prevention (US). Physical activity for everyone [Internet]. Atlanta (GA): Centers for Disease Control and Prevention (US); 2008 [reviewed 2008 24 Mar; updated 2008 Mar 26; cited 2008 Sep 22]. Available from: http://www.cdc.gov/nccdphp/dnpa/physical/everyone/health/index.htm
5. Centers for Disease Control and Prevention (US). Why should I be active? [Internet]. Atlanta (GA): Centers for Disease Control and Prevention (US); 2008 [cited 2008 Nov 20] Available from: http://www.cdc.gov/nccdphp/dnpa/physical/importance/why.htm
6. Cress ME, Buchner DM, Prohaska T, Rimmer J, Brown M, Macera C, DePietro L, Chodzko-Zajko W. Physical activity programs and behavioral counseling in older adult populations. Med Sci Sports Exer. 2004;36(11): 1997–2003.
7. Foster C, Wright G, Battista RA, Porcari JP. Training in the aging athlete. Curr Sports Med Rep. 2007 Mon;6(3):200–6.
8. Foley JP, editor. Jeffersonian cyclopedia. New York (NY): Russell and Russell; 1967. p. 402.
9. American heritage dictionary. 2nd college ed. Boston (MA): Houghton Mifflin; 1985.

CHAPTER 1

On Clinician Engagement and Counseling

Steven Jonas

INTRODUCTION: THE ESSENTIALS OF EXERCISE COUNSELING

The process known as exercise counseling is the central element in helping your patients to become regular exercisers and in providing them with an exercise prescription that will work for them. Many prescriptions that we clinicians provide—for medications, for various diagnostic procedures, and for various forms of non-medication therapy—are delivered *from* us *to* our patients. That is, they are "external" to the patient. Regular exercise, on the other hand, is an activity—a "therapy" if you will—that can be termed an "internal form of therapy," for it requires a major element of patient self-management. It is an intervention that your patient has to undertake himself or herself on an ongoing basis.

To effectively provide prescriptions for medications and other external forms of therapy, the highest levels of compliance are achieved when you are able to form a partnership with your patient. Yet doing so in these cases is not essential. Many patients willingly accept the clinician's direction and comply without entering into a partnership. With the exercise prescription, however—because its implementation requires an ongoing, active role for the patient—it is *essential* for effective counseling that a partnership be formed. You will help your patient get started, and you will provide advice as he or she goes along, on a when, as, and if basis. But, as noted, the *long-term* management in this case is primarily *self*-management. The patient will be in control. To help them take it and use it, you must be able work with them in a cooperative, rather than a totally directive, role.

Further differentiating regular exercise from most other health-promoting, disease-preventing, and disease treatment interventions is the fact that it takes *time* on an ongoing basis, time that was spent, before the person became a regular exerciser, doing something else. For as long one does it, it takes up time not formerly spent on it, but rather spent on other activities. Only a few other interventions—such as staying in an Alcoholics Anonymous or similar program for recovering alcoholics and other substance abusers or being on kidney dialysis—are similar. In contrast, consider the behavior of healthy eating.

Maintaining one's nutrition requires food shopping, food preparation, and eating. If a patient is currently practicing unhealthy eating habits and decides to convert to healthy ones, some time will be required to learn them. Some time may be spent in a weight-loss program, for example. However, eventually, if and when the nutritional goals the patient set are achieved, shopping/preparation/eating will take just about the same amount of time as before, perhaps even less. Thus, effective counseling for regular exercise has some special characteristics.

Foremost, as noted, to effectively implement the exercise prescription, the counseling process must take on the nature of a partnership. It cannot be a paternal/maternalistic relationship between clinician and patient. Especially with regular exercise, the "me doctor (or other clinician)/you patient," "do what I say to do [with perhaps a please attached]" will not work. Even though in the approach of Exercise is Medicine™ it comes in the form of a prescription, you are *asking* your patients, *suggesting* to them to do something that: a) will require the expenditure of time on regular basis, as noted; b) may well be totally foreign to them in terms of anything they have previously done in their lives; c) may at the beginning result in some mild pain (that is mild, not moderate-to-severe, if with your help they start off in the right way); d) may eventually require the expenditure of funds for anything from equipment to a gym membership; and e) in the minds of some will make them appear to be "different," not necessarily in a good way, to friends, family, and co-workers, as in the totally antihealth, "exercise nut" label.

Therefore, it is important to engage in interactive, rather than didactic, communication. You must be able to, or learn how to, exchange information with your patients rather than just deliver it to them. To be most effective, you will have to empower your patients to take control of the process, to learn for themselves, and, most important—as we will see in the following text and then throughout the book—to engage actively in the multiple steps in the health-promoting/positive-behavior-change process.

Let's begin with goal-setting. As a regional triathlon coaching organization, *Tri-Hard Sports Conditioning,* has said (1):

> There is much more to [regular exercise] than the physical aspects of conditioning. Training your mind is just as important and doing so begins with goal-setting. When a new athlete approaches us about coaching, the first thing we ask them is to tell us in detail about their goals. . . . When they write down their goals, they are forced to look at them and [consider them carefully]. This is important because . . . knowing what their goals are what motivates them to live well as they pursue [the achievement of them].

You will help your patients raise questions to which they can find the answers themselves, often in resources that you will either give them or direct them to. Actively finding those answers will produce much more effective learning than if you simply provide it for them directly. Of course you will provide certain answers of a didactic type: what is a good training regimen to get started with. But in most cases you will be much more effective if you help your patients find other kinds of answers for themselves, *e.g.,* what defines success for them.

Effective counseling for the regular exercise prescription requires that you be able to help your patients to mobilize their motivation. Chapters 4, 5, and 6 are devoted to presenting two different multistep approaches to the process. You and your patient will decide which one will likely work better for them, or it may be some combination of both. As we have noted and will continue to note on a regular basis, mobilizing motivation is the key to getting started and then to staying on course. Goal-setting is the central element in mobilizing motivation. Then, goal-evaluation/reassessment must take place on a regular basis if the motivation to continue as a regular exerciser is to be maintained. Furthermore, if the goals chosen are going to work for, not against, your patient, they must be realistic ones. They must be based on a definition of success for him or her that is realistic and achievable. Also, if they are going to work for your patient over the long-term, they must be "internal" goals, set for themselves, by themselves, not "external" ones, set with the hope of satisfying someone else.

IS COUNSELING FOR REGULAR EXERCISE EFFECTIVE?

The most recent (as of this writing) U.S. Preventive Services Task Force (USPSTF) recommendation on counseling for regular exercise was issued in 2002 (2). It concluded that: "there is insufficient evidence to determine whether counseling patients in primary care settings to promote physical activity leads to sustained increases in physical activity in adult patients." More recent controlled studies suggested that counseling for regular exercise in clinical practice may be effective in helping patients to become regular exercisers (3–5).

However, it is important to note that whatever the present evidence is for or against the effectiveness of exercise counseling by health care practitioners, the fact is that relatively few of you have received effective education and training in just how to do it so that it can work. Thus, to find that exercise counseling, by physicians at least, is not as effective as one would hope is not surprising, since only relatively few of them know how to do it effectively. Filling that unmet need for an education/training program in how to effectively provide the exercise prescription in clinical practice is of course the primary goal of Exercise is Medicine™. Finally, whether or not we know for sure that properly structured exercise counseling will work for **every** patient who needs it, certainly there are many—especially those who already have a positive attitude towards the subject—for whom, if correctly done, it will work. A central part of the Exercise is Medicine™ initiative, this book is intended to help you learn the knowledge, skills, and attitudes that will enable you to carry out these tasks effectively.

THE ROLE OF THE CLINICIAN

Your role in helping your patients to become and remain regular exercisers is obviously a complex one. Central to this is the element discussed above: helping your patients to mobilize their motivation, to set effective and realistic goals for themselves. Depending on your available time and interest, you may also help patients with the particulars of leisure-time scheduled exercise (LTSE, through The Scheduled Training Exercise Program [TSTEP]) that revolves around doing a sport or sports such as PaceWalking™ (our name for fast walking/power walking), running, cycling, swimming, the racquet sports, strength-training, the martial arts, the team sports, and so on and so forth. You may also help them in setting up effective exercise schedules for, or patterns of, lifestyle exercise (LE). As noted, this is exercise that is regularly incorporated into the activities of daily living, like climbing stairs instead of taking the elevator, walking to work if feasible, or parking in the far corner of the lot rather than circling around for a closer spot at the store or work. Lifestyle exercise has the advantage of being less time-intrusive than leisure-time scheduled exercise. Further, in certain settings it could even be time-conserving; for walking up a couple of flights of stairs may actually be quicker than waiting for the elevator.

For many clinicians, incorporating exercise promotion into one's practice is something new. There are some very simple approaches to providing the exercise prescription that you can undertake, and we will show how to do them, throughout the book. Some readers may want to delve into the matter more deeply, however. If you are one of them, there is a journey to be taken, parallel in a sense to that being taken by each patient who embarks on their own journey of regular exercise.

Other than those in an exercise-focused health profession such a physical therapy, few of us learned much, if anything, about regular exercise in either health sciences school or clinical training. If you are one of those who would like to get into the subject more deeply at some point down the road, there is a certain particular mind-set that you can develop, similar to the mind-set of the lifetime regular exerciser. You can be effective for your patients without going deeply into the subject. However, if you do want to get into the subject in some depth, we'll give you some guidelines for doing so, beginning in the next chapter. However, regardless of how deeply you want to get into the subject, it will be very helpful if you spend a bit of time thinking about goal-setting for yourself in your practice. The process will parallel the one the successful regular exerciser will have undertaken before they started down the regular-exercise pathway.

And so, you might want to think about such questions as: Why do I want to do this? Is exercise promotion important for my practice? Why? For which patients? What do I expect them to get out of it? What do I expect myself to get out it? That is, to avoid going off half-cocked and within a month giving up the whole idea, *carefully set your own goals.* The more certain you are of them, the more they make sense to you, the more convinced will you be that the whole enterprise is a good idea at whatever depth you initially set out to reach, the more certain will you be of your own commitment to it, and the better will be your own chances of success. For some readers, the journey will not only be one of incorporating regular exercise into their clinical practice, but also one of incorporating it into their own lives. If you are in this group, hopefully the practical program chapters in this book will be helpful for you in that endeavor too.

THE "THREE Ms" OF EFFECTIVE EXERCISE COUNSELING: MENTIONING, MODELING, MOTIVATING

Thus we come once again to the clinician's three principal roles in helping their patients to become regular exercisers. One is simple. Two are more complex. As noted in the Introduction, they are referred to as the "Three Ms," that is "Mentioning, Modeling, Motivating." For certain patients, those who are ready to get started trying to change a lifestyle behavior if given a slight push, just *mentioning* the advisability of regular exercise can be an effective intervention, just as mentioning losing weight or stopping the smoking of cigarettes can be very helpful for certain patients. You can *mention* regular exercise on a regular basis, at opportune times, when talking with patients about a wide variety of subjects. Without becoming a nag (a role you must avoid), you can make it clear to patients that you regard regular exercise as a good, very useful, health-promoting activity even if it is not on the patient's agenda at the present time. You simply have to a) remember to do it, and b) make a fairly quick judgment as to whether for that given patient mentioning is going to be helpful at that particular time.

Second, if you are so inclined, you can be a *model* for your patients by being or becoming a regular exerciser yourself. You will thus set an example for your patients. You will be able to recommend to them to do what you do as well as what you say. Perhaps of equal importance, whether you exercise at a minimum, modest, or robust level, you will be able to talk with your patients from experience. You will have firsthand knowledge of the difficulties of scheduling and will be able to share your own solutions to that problem. You will be able talk knowledgeably about technique and equipment for the sport(s) you do. You will be able to share how you make regular exercise fun, how you deal with safety, and how you handle both injury prevention and injury management. Finally, you will able to describe the benefits of regular exercise from personal experience.

Role modeling is not essential, but it is very helpful and highly recommended for several reasons. Most importantly, regularly exercising yourself, whether in the "lifestyle" or the "leisure-time scheduled" mode "shows the flag." It demonstrates to your patients that you have set exercise goals that make sense for you, and in one way or another you have made the time in your life to move towards them. Being able to talk from experience in working with a patient is also very helpful, whether that is the experience of the "lifestyle" or "leisure-time scheduled" modes. You know personally both the benefits and the difficulties of being a regular exerciser. You know how to focus, and you know that sometimes it can be difficult to maintain your focus. But you also know how to get it back and know all the benefits of getting it back and staying on track as a regular exerciser.

If you are currently inactive physically and decide to become a regular exerciser yourself, you will be able to share experiences that you have along the way with your patients—right from the start walking the same pathway that you are prescribing for them. If you are an athlete of one sort of another, you will be able to share sport-specific experiences with certain patients. It is not absolutely necessary for you to be a regular exerciser yourself in order to include the recommendation in your practice armamentarium, and you should not exclude it because you cannot or do not want to engage in the activity, at least at the present time. But if you do it, you will find it to be a great help in helping your patients, while at the same time reaping all of its benefits for yourself.

The third of the "Three Ms" is motivation, which just happens to be the most important element for getting started on the pathway to becoming a regular exerciser and then staying on it. How to help mobilize and maintain patient motivation is the process with which a major portion of this text (Chapters 4–6) is concerned. It is important to note here that as in any clinical approach to patient behavior change, in exercise counseling the role of the clinician is not to supply motivation to the patient. As discussed in detail in those chapters, effective motivation mobilization does not come from the outside. It comes from within, and it must be self-focused. However, you as a clinician have a very important role to play as the midwife, one might say, in helping patients to mobilize their own motivation, in the process "giving birth" as it were to a whole new aspect of their life.

To be most effective, you will be supportive, not instructive. You will by your own behavior reinforce the concept that effective motivation comes from within, that the patient's task is not to "find" it or acquire it outside of themselves. You will help your patient to understand that their task is to mobilize something that is already there in most people, to remove the internal roadblocks, not to worry about opening a new road from the outside in, as we will discuss in detail in those chapters below.

CONCLUSION

In helping patients to become regular exercisers, in providing the exercise prescription for them in ways that will work for them, there are a variety of roles that you can undertake, from fairly simple to fairly complex. One primary goal of this book is to help you choose a role in the whole process that is appropriate for you, at least at the time you are first reading this book. The aim is develop your new role so that you will find yourself being most helpful to your patients as they start down the pathway to becoming regular exercisers and then hopefully stay on it for the rest of their lives.

References

1. "USATNE Training Tips: Effective Goal Setting from Tri-Hard," http://www.tri-hard.com/, Jan., 2007.
2. U.S. Preventive Services Task Force. Guide to clinical preventive services. 3rd ed, Vol. 2, Chemoprevention and counseling. AHRQ Pub. No. 02-500. Rockville, MD: Agency for Healthcare Research and Quality; 2002. p. 53–8.
3. Petrella RJ, Koval JJ, Cunningham DA, Patterson DH. Can primary care doctors prescribe exercise to improve fitness? Am J Prev Med. 2003 May;24(4):316–22.
4. Elley CR, Kerse N, Arroll B, Robinson E. Effectiveness of counseling in patients on physical activity in general practice: cluster randomized controlled trial. BMJ, 2003 April; 326;793–9.
5. Pinto BM, Goldstein MG, Ashba J, Sciamanna CN, Jette A. Randomized controlled trial of physical activity counseling for older primary care patients. Am J Prev Med. 2005 November;29(4):247–55.

CHAPTER 2

On Organizing the Practice

Steven Jonas

INTRODUCTION

As we already have seen and will see in much more detail in the following chapters, in order to be successful in becoming regular exercisers, your patients will need to do a good deal of mental work before they start the physical activity. At the same time, if you are going to be successful in providing the exercise prescription in the way that will be most effective in helping your patients to achieve their goals, you will want to do some mental work as well. You will need to do a modest amount of it just to get going, more if you decide to get into the subject more deeply. Some of you will have already done that mental work. But many of you will not have. This chapter is about the thought processes you can engage in that will help you as you proceed down the road to organizing your practice and the way you practice to most effectively deliver the exercise prescription. We will start with some fairly simple approaches and proceed to some more complex ones.

USING THE "FIVE As" FRAMEWORK

One way of thinking about organizing both the way you work with individual patients and the way you manage your practice is to use what is called the "Five As Framework: Assess, Advise, Agree, Assist, Arrange follow-up" (1). You can use it in a step-wise fashion with patients, going along the pathway one step at a time. If you decide to undertake a reformulation of your practice, you can also use it comprehensively, as a planning model for doing so.

With patients in the first step, the *Assessment* process, you review both patient knowledge and present behavior(s). Hopefully, you will obtain some information about your patient's attitudes, beliefs, preferences, and feelings about the prospects of becoming a regular exerciser. Assessment can be carried out in a number of ways that we will discuss in more detail in Chapter 3, including use of pre-visit health risk appraisal instruments, questionnaires, and interactive computer-based systems.

Enabling you to effectively *Advise* your patients to accept the exercise pre-scription and implement it for themselves, in their own lives, is of course one of the central foci of this book. Advice is most effective when it is personal-ized and relates to your patient's particular situation. *Agreement* by the patient to engage in the process is the first step that they need to take in order to get on the pathway of exercising regularly. As noted, actively *Assisting* the patient to engage in the activity is a role that clinicians have in implementing few other prescriptions. In this case, because of the ongoing nature of the behav-ior change process that is at the center of becoming a regular exerciser, it is necessary for the clinician to be proactive. Your ongoing help is essential if your patients are going to build up their confidence in their own ability to actually effect the necessary behavior change(s).

Arrange here refers to arrangements that your patient will be making, from scheduling, to choosing the type(s) of regular exercise they are going to engage in, to finding locations, acquiring equipment, learning new sport(s) if applicable, and so on and so forth. It also refers to arrangements that you will be making, that is, if this is a new function for your practice or if you will be considerably expanding your focus on it, and to arranging to engage in long-term follow-up with your patients.

CREATING AND USING THE PHYSICIAN/ FITNESS–PROFESSIONAL TEAM

As part of what can help you to become effective, we turn to a consideration of creating, being part of, and using the physician–fitness professional team, as developed by the American College of Sports Medicine itself. The ACSM recognizes, trains, and certifies a broad range of Fitness Professionals. In addi-tion to them, there are numerous other recognized health professionals, described briefly in the following paragraphs, dealing with regular exercise and regular exercisers, present or potential. The list includes: the physical therapist, the occupational therapist, the athletic trainer, the chiropractor, the sports psychologist, the health educator, the nutritionist, the addiction coun-selor, the social worker, and the certified athletic trainer.

In dealing with one or another aspect of regular exercise for one patient or another, clinicians making referrals to other clinicians obviously have a wide range of potential colleagues to choose from. The choice for referral, when made, should reflect the needs of the particular patient in question. All of these healthcare professionals can be part of the regular-exercise-promoting team. In some locales certain of them may sit under one roof. Or they may form a "vir-tual team," working in different locations but working together and commu-nicating regularly about individual patients, the interventions they are using, and new developments they come across.

The ACSM's *Guidelines for Exercise Testing and Prescription,* now in its 8th edition (GETP8), provides a more in-depth, detailed approach to screening patients, exercise testing protocols, and exercise prescription. This text is highly recommended to exercise professionals and the interested clinician. The balance of this section of this chapter is drawn from the text of the Report of the Guidelines for Exercise Testing and Prescription, 8th edition, Appendix D (2).

The first ACSM clinical certification was initiated over 30 years ago in conjunction with the publication of the first edition of the GETP. That era was marked by, first, the rapid development of exercise programs for patients with stable coronary artery disease (CAD). ACSM sought a means to disseminate accurate information on this healthcare initiative through the expression of consensus from its members in basic science, clinical practice, and education. Thus, these early clinical certifications were viewed as an aid to the establishment of safe and scientifically based exercise services within the framework of cardiac rehabilitation practice as it was then understood.

The ongoing development of the health/fitness certifications in the 1980s reflected ACSM's intent to increase the availability of qualified professionals to provide scientifically sound advice and supervision regarding appropriate physical activities for health maintenance in the apparently healthy adult population. Since 1975, more than 35,000 certificates have been awarded in the several ACSM certification categories. With this consistent growth, ACSM has taken steps to ensure that its competency-based certifications will continue to be regarded as the premier set of programs in the exercise field.

The principal Fitness Professionals recognized by ACSM are as follows. All should be considered when a Physician–Fitness Professional team is being developed. If they are ACSM-certified, one can be assured that their education will have been based upon a common body of Knowledge, Skills, and Attitudes (KSAs), with the appropriate specializations for each of the professions.

The ACSM Certified Personal Trainer℠ is a fitness professional involved in developing and implementing an individualized approach to exercise leadership in healthy populations and/or those individuals with medical clearance to exercise. Using a variety of teaching techniques, the ACSM Certified Personal Trainer℠ is proficient in leading and demonstrating safe and effective methods of exercise by applying the fundamental principles of exercise science. The ACSM Certified Personal Trainer℠ is familiar with forms of exercise used to improve, maintain, and/or optimize health-related components of physical fitness and performance. The ACSM Certified Personal Trainer℠ is proficient in writing appropriate exercise recommendations, leading and demonstrating safe and effective methods of exercise, and motivating individuals to begin and to continue with their healthy behaviors.

The ACSM Health/Fitness Instructor® (HFI) is a health and fitness professional holding a degree qualified for career pursuits in the university, corporate, commercial, hospital, and community settings. The HFI has knowledge and skills in management, administration, training, and supervising entry-level personnel. The HFI is skilled in conducting risk stratification, conducting physical fitness assessments and interpreting results, constructing appropriate exercise prescriptions and motivating apparently healthy individuals and individuals with medically-controlled diseases to adopt and maintain healthy lifestyle behaviors

The ACSM Exercise Specialist® (ES) is a healthcare professional certified by ACSM to deliver a variety of exercise assessment, training, rehabilitation, risk factor identification, and lifestyle management services to individuals with or at risk for cardiovascular, pulmonary, and metabolic disease(s). These services are typically delivered in cardiovascular/pulmonary rehabilitation programs, physicians' offices, or medical fitness centers. The ACSM Exercise Specialist® is also competent to provide exercise-related consulting for research, public health, and other clinical and non-clinical services and programs.

The ACSM Registered Clinical Exercise Physiologist® (RCEP) is an allied health professional who works in the application of physical activity and behavioral interventions for those clinical conditions where they have been shown to provide therapeutic and/or functional benefit. Persons for whom RCEP services are appropriate may include, but are not limited to, those individuals with cardiovascular, pulmonary, metabolic, orthopedic, musculoskeletal, neuromuscular, neoplastic, immunologic, or hematologic disease. The RCEP provides primary and secondary prevention strategies designed to improve fitness and health in populations ranging from children to older adults. The RCEP performs exercise screening, exercise and fitness testing, exercise prescription, exercise and physical activity counseling, exercise supervision, exercise and health education/promotion, and measurement and evaluation of exercise- and physical activity-related outcome measures. The RCEP works individually or as part of an interdisciplinary team in a clinical, community, or public health setting. The practice and supervision of the RCEP is guided by published professional guidelines, standards, and applicable state and federal regulations.

Certification at a given level requires the candidate to have a knowledge and skills base commensurate with that specific level of certification. In addition, the HFI level of certification incorporates the KSAs associated with the ACSM Certified Personal Trainer℠ certification; the ES level of certification incorporates the KSAs associated with the CPT and HFI certification; and the RCEP level of certification incorporates the KSAs associated with the CPT, HFI, and ES levels of certification. In addition, each level of certification has minimum requirements for experience, level of education, or other certifications.

So, whatever type of clinician you are, you are not alone in venturing into effectively providing the exercise prescription for your patients. At least you don't have to be.

ORGANIZING THE PRACTICE

The myriad details of this topic could fill a whole chapter. Rather than presenting all of them here, we are going to briefly consider the various elements that you will be considering to a greater or lesser extent, depending upon how "organized" you decide to become.

Activity Level As a Vital Sign: Noting, Recording, and Reminding

In a practice organized to regularly prescribe regular exercise, given its role in achieving and maintaining a state of good health (see Chapter 1), your patients' physical activity status should be considered as a vital sign to be measured regularly. As such, while other vital signs such as blood pressure and pulse are being taken, staff should ask if the patient is physically active, at least at a moderate intensity at least 30 minutes per day, five days per week. Appropriate notation on the patient's paper or electronic medical record will call your attention to those inactive patients who most need your counseling to begin a program of physical activity. Patients who are already physically active can be encouraged to maintain, or if indicated, increase their exercise level. Reminders for clinicians, patients, and other staff can include stickers, patient logs, and nurse follow-up calls, as indicated. Similar interventions have led to relative success in the practice of clinicians prescribing smoking cessation.

Personnel

As noted above, there is obviously a very broad range of personnel that can provide one or more of the elements of exercise counseling and indeed can provide the exercise prescription (since it is a prescription that one does not have to, or is legally empowered to provide). If you are in a solo practice, you are obviously going to choose which elements you are going to include in your own approach to providing the exercise prescription. If you have staff working with and/or for you, as in a medical office, you are going to have to figure how the various responsibilities are going to be distributed among them. That process will work best, of course, if you bring your staff into the decision-making process. If you are part of a group of practitioners providing the same service, as in a physical therapy practice, together you will decide who does what for whom. In a large multi-specialty medical group practice you may have the luxury of having health professionals other than physicians on staff, such as a health educator, a social worker, a clinical psychologist, an athletic trainer, who can take major parts of the patient education functions for regular exerciser, according to a plan that is jointly set up.

Charging, What to Charge, and Billing

This can be a toughie. Since few clinicians provide exercise counseling sessions now, fee-setting will involve much guesswork, much trial-and-error, and much finding out both how much it costs your practice and how much the traffic will bear. Although exercise counseling per se, at least for a limited number of sessions, may in the future be a covered service under national health reform, presently not too many insurance plans cover it. You may decide to get into providing more extensive exercise counseling yourself, on a fee-for-service basis. If so, you will have to decide how long the sessions will be, how many of them will comprise a package, what you will cover, and what you will charge (given that most patients will be paying for the service out-of-pocket). In a group practice setting, if the practice is large enough, you may have a staff member to whom you will be able to assign responsibility for this function, again setting a standard fee for a standard package of services.

This all being said, an important piece of the ACSM's Exercise is Medicine™ program's agenda is to achieve the provision of appropriate reimbursement from third-party payors for clinicians counseling their patients about physical activity and providing exercise prescriptions. Unfortunately there is not yet (as of 2008) a formal ICD-9 code reflecting sedentary behavior, such as what might be called the *"Exercise Deficit Disorder (EDD)."* In the interim, clinicians can code and bill Medicare (and certain other insurance carriers as they exercise their choices in this matter) for the *additional* time spent in counseling patients about physical activity and exercise, as long as the clinician clearly reports the *medical* indication for the services rendered (3). That is (as of the time of writing), Medicare does not allow billing "by time" for preventive services. Nor does it allow for writing and delivering an exercise prescription *per se*. However, patients who need this type of counseling often present with a chronic medical problem with mild exacerbation. For a summary, see the Three-Minute Drill 2-1. The CPT (Current Procedural Terminology) for this (as of 2008) is 99213: "Established Visit Office Patient." In addition, there

THREE-MINUTE DRILL, 2 – 1

- Medicare does not reimburse "by time" for preventive services so the underlying medical indication must be clearly stated.
- Medicare will not reimburse for providing an exercise prescription, but time spent counseling your patient about physical activity may help support billing "by time."
- The extra time needs to be reported as the portion of the total time spent in the encounter.
- **EXAMPLE:** "In this 25 minute visit the majority of the time was spent in face-to-face counseling and coordinating care concerned with the patient's medical condition (e.g., obesity, hypertension, etc.), including counseling on physical activity."

is CPT 99214, which covers chronic problems requiring diagnostic tests for management or dealing with a mild exacerbation. The list of chronic problems coming under these codes may include obesity, hypertension, arthritis, hyperlipidemia, etc.

Further, rather than being limited to reporting CPT 99213, because of the nature of the presenting problems most frequently associated with "EDD," a physician may bill CPT 99214 if the total visit interval is ≥ 25 min, or CPT 99215 if the total visit interval is ≥ 40 min. When a physician bills "by time," the total visit interval drives the level billed. That is, the limiting effect of the nature of the presenting problem(s) is replaced by: 1) documentation of the total visit interval; 2) attestation that the majority of the visit was for counseling and coordinating care; and 3) documentation of the topics discussed lending credibility to the interval reported.

Setting Up Evening Groups

There have been reports by office-based practitioners of success with exercise groups, meeting one evening a week, for a modest fee per person. Psychotherapists, of course, have extensive experience with patient groups. It does take some time to organize this kind of activity. But once it is done, this form for counseling can be very productive for both you and your patients. It is efficient, and if the fee structure is set correctly, it can be cost-effective for you. For the patients who come to it, it not only provides for the learning experience, but there is also the element of peer input and support in dealing with commonly experienced problems and challenges.

Active Living Every Day (http://www.activeliving.info/) is an organized program based on research from the Cooper Institute. It trains facilitators to lead 20 weekly group sessions guiding patients from inactivity to the minimal levels of recommended activity. You or a member of your staff can be trained as a facilitator.

Using Written Materials

It will be useful to have written materials available for your patients. First, there are the "Three Minute Drills" and other tables in this book that you may find helpful. Second, resources for clinicians, educators, ACSM certified professionals, the general public, the media, researchers, speakers, sponsors, and students can all be found at the ACSM website (www.acsm.org). Third, free handouts may be available from your local and/or state health department, the local chapter of a voluntary agency like the American Heart Association, from several Federal government agencies, including the United States Public Health Service's Office of Disease Prevention and Health Promotion, the Federal Centers for Disease Control and Prevention, and the President's Council on Physical Fitness and Sport, and from certain health and fitness professional organizations (see Appendix II, Resources, for suggested organizations, with URLs). Magazines can be helpful, and you may want to recommend one or more of them (also see Appendix II).

You can also provide patients with a list of recommended books that can be purchased at local bookstores and on the Web, starting with the *ACSM Fitness Book* (4). To go further than it, you will have to spend some time at least looking at some of the other sources listed in the Resource List, and others that may catch your eye, and periodically you will have to check on availability. If you are in a practice setting in which items are sold to patients at retail, you may want to offer one or more books for sale directly to them.

Using Community Resources

There is a wide variety of community resources that may be available for use by patients engaging in scheduled regular exercise, depending upon where they live. They include health clubs and gyms (both of which may have, among many other facilities, swimming pools); free-standing swimming pools; tracks (such as at the local high school that may be available for community use at certain times of the day, during certain seasons of the year); bike routes, either dedicated or laid on the public roads; walking/running roads, paths and trails; tennis and basketball courts; community-based recreation centers, shopping malls that have pre- and/or post-opening walking programs, and multipurpose sports clubs.

Some community facilities are free and some cost money, from a little for an annual membership in a local cycling club to what can be a lot, depending the deal one is able to make, for a health club/gym/YMCA/YMHA/JCC (Jewish Community Center)/church-based exercise club membership. All of the above do/may have facilities that can range from the very simple to the highly sophisticated. Although not every clinician has the time or inclination to do so, it can be very helpful for you to spend some time learning about and evaluating the available resources in your community. Making that time investment up front can in the long run save you a great deal of time in working with your patients and provide important substantive assistance for them. Further, if you have the time and the inclination, you could consider setting up formal referral relationships with one or more community resources, as appropriate. You might even be able to work out a formal arrangement with a fee-based sports/exercise club where you could derive some tangible benefit from making successful referrals.

Free are such venues as the local high school (and in some cases the local college) track and swimming pool. For the latter, there are often community-times set, and while they might not be at the most convenient hours, and the lap lanes may be fairly full, use is at least free or available for a very modest fee. Also free are designated walking/running/cycling trails in parks and green-belts. The local government recreation office, state and local parks departments, as well as certain state and local health departments can be very helpful in locating facilities. Some university and high school gymnasiums have facilities open to the general public at certain hours. There are also specialized facilities open to the public for a fee, such as racquet-ball clubs. As for tennis, many communities have courts available, either free or for a modest fee. There may be a variety of individual membership sports associations and clubs, such as for Masters swimming, walking, running, cycling, skiing, triathlon, racquet sports, and team sports. Information will be available on many of these kinds of facilities and organizations from your local government recreation office, specialized and general sporting good stores, and on the web.

THINKING ABOUT IT AS A CLINICIAN: YOUR OWN BEHAVIOR CHANGE PROCESS

To become regular exercisers, your patients will need to go through a process of behavior change that we discuss in detail in Chapters 4–6. As noted above, there is much that you can do fairly quickly and fairly simply to begin incorporating the provision of the exercise prescription as a regular part of your practice. However, if you want to get into the subject at greater depth, you may find that you will, at some level, go through something of a *professional* behavior change process. In this section we provide a guide for those of you who would like to give it a try. It is a behavior change process that, interestingly enough, is very similar to what your patients will go through on their way to successfully becoming regular exercisers.

Foremost, just like any patient setting out to engage in a health-promoting behavior change of one sort or another, you will have to mobilize your motivation to do it. You will have to mobilize resources; you will have to find and make the time; you will have to convince colleagues; you will have to provide leadership. Developing and implementing a plan for incorporating counseling for the regular exercise prescription into your practice, is perhaps best approached by answering a series of questions for yourself. We think that it is most appropriate that we conclude this chapter with these questions, in Table 2.1. Just as becoming and staying a regular exerciser is not always easy, becoming and staying as a regular provider of the regular exercise prescription is also not always easy. Hopefully, this list of questions will help you to organize your own thinking about the enterprise. Hopefully, the further information in this book will then equip you to take on this task and to achieve success in it. If you are able to do so, we are confident that you will then be able to effectively help your patients to take on the task of regularly exercising.

TABLE 2.1 Clinician Self-Assessment: Including the
Exercise Prescription in Your Practice

1. Is providing the exercise prescription for my patients important in my practice? How important is it? In other words, as I contemplate adding the exercise prescription to my clinical armamentarium, what are my own goals for doing so?

2. As part of my own goal-setting process, let me think about why is it important for *me* to do this now, at this stage of my career, in my practice as it is currently set up.

3. What do I think is missing in my practice currently that makes me think about doing something new? Why do I think that?

4. For which patients am I thinking about doing this? All of them? Some of them? How will I make my choices in this regard? How will I engage my patients in that decision-making process?

5. If my practice is bigger than just me and especially if I am not the only decision-maker, I will have to think more broadly. That is, once I have established my goals for myself, I should likely think about what goals I would like to see adopted for my practice. Once I have decided to change my own practice behavior, will I be able to work with my colleagues to help them change theirs, and is that necessary?

6. Is role-modeling (as discussed above) important for my patients? If so, by whom? What does this mean for me? Do I want to invest my personal time in this? If I am not already a regular exerciser and have decided to become one, what are my own goals for doing so and just what is it that I am going to do? "Lifestyle exercise"? "Leisure-time scheduled"? For either, how am I going to find the time/make the time? What is it exactly that I am going to do?

7. If I think that there is material to learn here, how much time do I want to invest in doing so? In terms of the specifics, how should I go about learning them, incorporating them into my own base of knowledge and skills?

8. If I am in charge of the practice, who should do the counseling for the exercise prescription? Myself? Members of my staff? Somebody new whom I might bring in part-time, like a physical therapist, a health/fitness professional, or a health educator? If one or more of us is going to need some education and training, how is that going to be provided and who is going to do it? (Hopefully, this book will be enough, but you may have to go beyond it.)

9. Whoever does the counseling for the exercise prescription, how is the function going to be paid for? Do I charge patients for this service? If so, how and how much? How can I arrange for health insurance reimbursement?

10. Do I want to try using patient groups for exercise promotion? If so, how are they going to be organized, who is going to lead them, how are they going to be paid (if they are), and how are we going to charge our patients (if we do)?

11. What about making use of community resources?

12. How much time am I willing to invest in developing an exercise promotion component in my practice? If not I, then who?

References

1. Glasgow RE, Goldstein MG. Introduction to the principles of health behavior change. In: Woolf SH, Jonas S, Kaplan-Liss E, editors. Health promotion and disease prevention in clinical practice. 2nd ed. Philadelphia, PA: Lippincott Williams and Wilkins; 2008. p. 134–9.
2. American College of Sports Medicine. ACSM's guidelines for exercise testing and prescription. 8th ed. Philadelphia: Lippincott Williams & Wilkins; 2009. p. 2–11.
3. CMS IOM Manual: Section 30.6—Evaluation and Management Service Codes, General (Codes 99201–99499); C. Selection of Level of Evaluation and Management Service Based on Duration of Coordination of Care and/or Counseling. http://www.cms.hhs.gov/manuals/downloads/clm104c12.pdf.
4. American College of Sports Medicine. ACSM fitness book. 3rd ed. Champaign, IL: Human Kinetics; 2003. 175 p.

CHAPTER 3

Risk Assessment and Exercise Screening

Edward M. Phillips and Jennifer Capell

INTRODUCTION

Beginning the Exercise Prescription Process

As discussed in Chapters 1 and 2, regular physical activity in the form of lifestyle exercise or leisure-time scheduled exercise confers numerous health benefits to the participants. As such, the public health goal for all adults to accumulate 30 minutes of moderate physical activity at least five days per week or to engage in 20 minutes of vigorous exercise at least three days per week is of paramount importance (1). Now that you are more engaged in the importance of counseling your patients to become physically active and to maintain their exercise programs, the question of safety to exercise arises.

Because of the overwhelming benefits of exercise, the universal hazards of inactivity, and the relatively rare serious side effects of exercise, the screening process should not present a burden to the clinician or prevent patients from initiating light- or moderate-intensity physical activity. (See Chapter 8 for discussion of exercise intensity.)

For the vast majority of your patients, the information that you as a clinician already possess about their medical history is sufficient to screen for safety to begin or increase exercise. This information includes a medical history of cardiac, pulmonary, and metabolic disease; known cardiac risk factors; signs and symptoms elicited during a routine physical examination and simple probing about their current level of activity—"are you physically active, at a moderate intensity at least 30 minutes per day, 5 times per week?" This question may be elicited as a "vital sign" at the clinical encounter to determine the need for your patient to initiate, increase, or continue physical activity.

In this chapter, we provide you with a systematic method of assessing your patient's medical status to reduce the chance that your patient may risk injury or illness (particularly to his or her heart) by exercising. As you will see, almost all patients will benefit from exercise, but some, especially those patients with known disease, signs and symptoms, or risk factors for cardiovascular, pulmonary, or metabolic disease, may need to have certain modifications or restrictions placed on their exercise program.

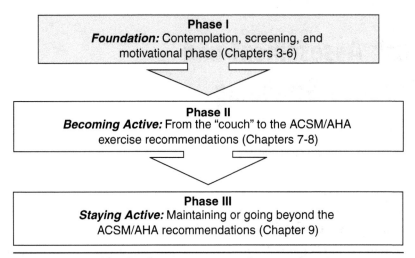

Figure 3.1 • Lifestyle Changes: From Sedentary to Active

From there the more challenging aspects of mobilizing your patient's motivation will follow. The combination of the assessment and evaluation of your patient's safety to exercise and mobilizing motivation constitutes the Foundation Phase of the exercise prescription (Figure 3.1).

The process of making lifestyle changes from sedentary to active is a slow, but important aspect of your patient's health. It is our hope that you will play an effective role in this healthy transformation. As you progress through this book, you will see that the process of prescribing exercise to your patient involves numerous stages before actually giving your patient the exercise prescription. In fact, we do not cover the prescription until Chapter 8. The preliminary stages in this process are crucial. As Figure 3.1 illustrates, this process begins with the Foundation Phase, in which patients need to be psychologically and motivationally ready to begin making lifestyle changes toward a more active routine. These subjects are covered fully in Chapters 4–6.

Risks of Sedentary Behavior

Before we present the possible risks of exercise, let's begin with the question: "Is this patient safe to remain sedentary?" In most instances remaining inactive will harm the patient. Sedentary behavior is identified by the American Heart Association as a distinct cardiovascular risk factor (2) with prevalence twice that of smoking, hypertension, and dyslipidemia. While there are relatively rare serious risks to beginning an exercise program, there are universal risks from inactivity. Table 3.1 illustrates some of the risks associated with a sedentary lifestyle.

TABLE 3.1 Risks of Sedentary Behavior

Reduced functional capacity	
Osteoporosis	
Obesity	
Anxiety and depression	Hypertension
Cardiovascular disease	Colon cancer
Thromboembolic stroke	Breast cancer
Type 2 diabetes mellitus	

Kesaniemi et al. Med. Sci. Sport Exerc. 33(6 Suppl):S531–S538, 2001.

Risks of Exercise

Continuing with our prevailing metaphor of using exercise as a medication to promote health as well as to prevent and treat illness, let us now explore the potential risks from using this "medicine" and present an effective and efficient means to mitigate these risks. Just as clinicians are aware of the risks or side effects of a prescribed medication, you must also be aware of the risks and side effects from prescribing physical activity. The risks of participation in exercise range from the most common—muscle soreness and musculoskeletal injury (please see discussion in Chapter 7)—to the most serious—myocardial infarctions and sudden cardiac death (3). Our primary focus in this chapter is on cardiovascular risks.

Cardiovascular Risks Associated with Exercise

Vigorous physical activity has been shown to acutely increase the risk of sudden cardiac death and myocardial infarction among individuals with both diagnosed and occult cardiac conditions (3). Further, atherosclerotic coronary artery disease is the overwhelming cause of exercise-related deaths in adults, accounting for one exertion-related death per year for every 15,000–18,000 seemingly healthy men (3). The relative risk of both exercise-related myocardial infarction and sudden death is most likely in individuals who are the least physically active and who engage in unaccustomed vigorous physical activity (3). Therefore, sedentary adults should avoid unaccustomed vigorous activity—they should begin with low- or moderate-intensity exercise and gradually increase their activity levels over time (3) (Chapters 7–10 detail the appropriate progression of exercise to mitigate these risks).

Even amongst patients with known cardiac disease undergoing cardiac rehabilitation programs, the incidence of adverse cardiac events are rare: cardiac arrest = 1:117,000; nonfatal myocardial infarction = 1:220,000; and death = 1:750,000 patient-hours of participation (3).

Purposes of Screening

As with any "medication," the risks or side effects can be minimized through appropriate prescription and progression. Therefore, appropriate screening of patients must be undertaken before beginning or increasing physical activity levels. The risk factors to be considered include cardiovascular, pulmonary, and metabolic conditions as well as specific conditions such as pregnancy, old age, osteoporosis, and others that we consider in depth in Chapter 13.

As we have just illustrated, in the vast majority of patients, the benefits of exercise far outweigh the serious risks of exercise and the universal risks of remaining sedentary. Further, by knowing your patient's specific medical history, symptoms, and disease risk factors, and modifying his exercise program accordingly, you can further decrease his risk of suffering from an exercise-induced cardiac event. The health screening process that we describe in this chapter enables your patient to be assessed in a systematic manner to determine his risk level for adverse medical events when exercising. While prudent screening is warranted for patients initiating, continuing, or advancing their exercise programs, this process should not present a barrier to participation in physical activity.

As the clinician, the algorithms presented in this chapter will help to identify factors that may 1) require preparticipation medical screening or exercise testing; 2) warrant a clinically or professionally supervised program or limitations on the intensity at which a patient is safe to exercise; or 3) (in a small number of patients) may exclude your patient from participation. Your responsibility is to follow a logical and practical sequence to acquire health information, assess risk, and provide the exercise prescription with appropriate precautions to your patient.

RISK ASSESSMENT

Self-Assessment

Patients may screen themselves to determine if a formal medical assessment is warranted by following the recommendation of the Surgeon Generals' Report on Physical Activity and Health (1996): "previously inactive men over age 40 and women over age 50, and people at high risk for cardiovascular disease (CVD) should first consult a physician before embarking on a program of vigorous physical activity to which they are unaccustomed" (4). Please note the emphasis on the *vigorous* intensity. Initiating moderate-intensity physical activity does not require this screening.

Alternatively, the patient may also use a self-guided questionnaire such as the Physical Activity Readiness Questionnaire (PAR-Q; Figure 3.2). This self-guided, 7-question screening tool quickly identifies patients with conditions or risk factors that require further assessment before commencing an

Physical Activity Readiness
Questionnaire - PAR-Q
(revised 2002)

PAR-Q & YOU

(A Questionnaire for People Aged 15 to 69)

Regular physical activity is fun and healthy, and increasingly more people are starting to become more active every day. Being more active is very safe for most people. However, some people should check with their doctor before they start becoming much more physically active.

If you are planning to become much more physically active than you are now, start by answering the seven questions in the box below. If you are between the ages of 15 and 69, the PAR-Q will tell you if you should check with your doctor before you start. If you are over 69 years of age, and you are not used to being very active, check with your doctor.

Common sense is your best guide when you answer these questions. Please read the questions carefully and answer each one honestly: check YES or NO.

YES	NO	
☐	☐	**1. Has your doctor ever said that you have a heart condition and that you should only do physical activity recommended by a doctor?**
☐	☐	**2. Do you feel pain in your chest when you do physical activity?**
☐	☐	**3. In the past month, have you had chest pain when you were not doing physical activity?**
☐	☐	**4. Do you lose your balance because of dizziness or do you ever lose consciousness?**
☐	☐	**5. Do you have a bone or joint problem (for example, back, knee or hip) that could be made worse by a change in your physical activity?**
☐	☐	**6. Is your doctor currently prescribing drugs (for example, water pills) for your blood pressure or heart condition?**
☐	☐	**7. Do you know of <u>any other reason</u> why you should not do physical activity?**

If

you

answered

YES to one or more questions

Talk with your doctor by phone or in person BEFORE you start becoming much more physically active or BEFORE you have a fitness appraisal. Tell your doctor about the PAR-Q and which questions you answered YES.

- You may be able to do any activity you want — as long as you start slowly and build up gradually. Or, you may need to restrict your activities to those which are safe for you. Talk with your doctor about the kinds of activities you wish to participate in and follow his/her advice.
- Find out which community programs are safe and helpful for you.

NO to all questions

If you answered NO honestly to all PAR-Q questions, you can be reasonably sure that you can:

- start becoming much more physically active — begin slowly and build up gradually. This is the safest and easiest way to go.
- take part in a fitness appraisal — this is an excellent way to determine your basic fitness so that you can plan the best way for you to live actively. It is also highly recommended that you have your blood pressure evaluated. If your reading is over 144/94, talk with your doctor before you start becoming much more physically active.

DELAY BECOMING MUCH MORE ACTIVE:

- if you are not feeling well because of a temporary illness such as a cold or a fever — wait until you feel better; or
- if you are or may be pregnant — talk to your doctor before you start becoming more active.

PLEASE NOTE: If your health changes so that you then answer YES to any of the above questions, tell your fitness or health professional. Ask whether you should change your physical activity plan.

Informed Use of the PAR-Q: The Canadian Society for Exercise Physiology, Health Canada, and their agents assume no liability for persons who undertake physical activity, and if in doubt after completing this questionnaire, consult your doctor prior to physical activity.

No changes permitted. You are encouraged to photocopy the PAR-Q but only if you use the entire form.

NOTE: If the PAR-Q is being given to a person before he or she participates in a physical activity program or a fitness appraisal, this section may be used for legal or administrative purposes.

"I have read, understood and completed this questionnaire. Any questions I had were answered to my full satisfaction."

NAME _____

SIGNATURE _____   DATE_____

SIGNATURE OF PARENT _____   WITNESS _____
or GUARDIAN (for participants under the age of majority)

Note: This physical activity clearance is valid for a maximum of 12 months from the date it is completed and becomes invalid if your condition changes so that you would answer YES to any of the seven questions.

CSEP
SCPE © Canadian Society for Exercise Physiology   Supported by: 🍁   Health   Santé   continued on other side...
Canada   Canada

Figure 3.2 • Physical Activity Readiness Questionnaire (PAR-Q).

Source: *Physical Activity Readiness Questionnaire (PAR-Q)* © 2002. Used with permission from the Canadian Society for Exercise Physiology, www.csep.ca.

(continued)

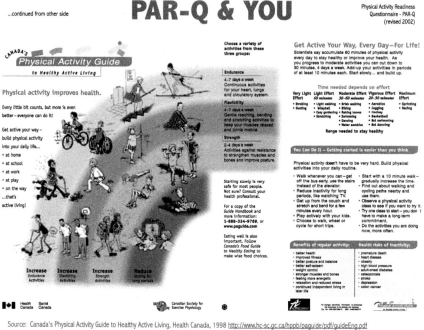

Source: Canada's Physical Activity Guide to Healthy Active Living, Health Canada, 1998 http://www.hc-sc.gc.ca/hppb/paguide/pdf/guideEng.pdf
© Reproduced with permission from the Minister of Public Works and Government Services Canada, 2002.

FITNESS AND HEALTH PROFESSIONALS MAY BE INTERESTED IN THE INFORMATION BELOW:

The following companion forms are available for doctors' use by contacting the Canadian Society for Exercise Physiology (address below):

The **Physical Activity Readiness Medical Examination (PARmed-X)** — to be used by doctors with people who answer YES to one or more questions on the PAR-Q.

The **Physical Activity Readiness Medical Examination for Pregnancy (PARmed-X for Pregnancy)** — to be used by doctors with pregnant patients who wish to become more active.

References:
Arraix, G.A., Wigle, D.T., Mao, Y. (1992). Risk Assessment of Physical Activity and Physical Fitness in the Canada Health Survey Follow-Up Study. **J. Clin. Epidemiol.** 45:4 419-428.
Mottola, M., Wolfe, L.A. (1994). Active Living and Pregnancy, In: A. Quinney, L. Gauvin, T. Wall (eds.), **Toward Active Living: Proceedings of the International Conference on Physical Activity, Fitness and Health.** Champaign, IL: Human Kinetics.
PAR-Q Validation Report, British Columbia Ministry of Health, 1978.
Thomas, S., Reading, J., Shephard, R.J. (1992). Revision of the Physical Activity Readiness Questionnaire (PAR-Q). **Can. J. Spt. Sci.** 17:4 338-345.

Figure 3.2 • (*Continued*)

exercise program. The PAR-Q is available online (at www.csep.ca), so your patients can complete the PAR-Q independently; however, you may find it beneficial to have patients fill out the questionnaire while waiting for their appointment with you. If your patient answers *no* to all 7 questions, he is at a LOW RISK for health complications, and is generally safe to begin an exercise program without supervision at any intensity. Additional tools such as the AHA/ACSM Health/Fitness Facility Preparticipation Screening Questionnaire (See Appendix) will effectively direct appropriate patients for further evaluation. Either of these tools can be completed upon planned entry to a fitness facility or as part of their appointment with you.

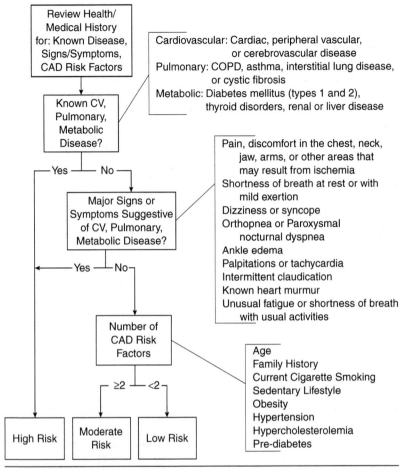

Figure 3.3 • Risk Stratification of Patients (From ACSM's guidelines for exercise testing and prescription. 8th ed. Philadelphia: Lippincott Williams & Wilkins; 2009.)

Screening Guidelines

The algorithm presented in Figure 3.3 and Table 3.2 outline the screening process that you will go through to determine your patient's risk level. This assessment process has been designed based on the eighth edition of ACSM's *Guidelines for Exercise Testing and Prescription*. Both the authors of this book and the ACSM (5) recognize "guidelines for risk stratification published by other organizations such as the American Heart Association (AHA) [6–9] and the American Association of Cardiovascular and Pulmonary Rehabilitation (AACVPR)." [10] They recommend that "[e]xercise and health/fitness professionals should also be familiar with these other guidelines when establishing

TABLE 3.2 Medical History, Signs and Symptoms, and Risk Factors for Risk Stratification

Cardiovascular, Pulmonary, or Metabolic Disease (HIGH RISK):

Cardiovascular disease (CVD):
- cardiac disease
- peripheral artery disease (PAD)
- cerebrovascular disease
- heart attack or heart failure
- heart surgery or transplantation
- cardiac catheterization
- coronary angioplasty
- heart valve disease
- congenital heart disease
- pacemaker/implantable cardiac defibrillator

Metabolic disease:
- diabetes mellitus (type 1 or 2)
- renal or liver disease
- thyroid disorders

Pulmonary disease:
- chronic obstructive pulmonary disease
- asthma
- interstitial lung disease
- cystic fibrosis

Major Signs and Symptoms of Cardiovascular, Pulmonary or Metabolic Disease (HIGH RISK):

- chest discomfort with exertion
- dizziness, fainting or blackouts
- heart rhythm disturbance
- taking heart medications
- bilateral ankle edema
- unreasonable breathlessness (at rest, with mild exercise, or when recumbent)
- burning or cramping sensation in lower legs when walking short distances
- pain or discomfort in the chest, neck, jaw, arms, or elsewhere that may be due to ischemia

Cardiovascular, Pulmonary or Metabolic Risk Factors: (<2 risk factors = LOW RISK; ≥2 = MODERATE RISK):

- male > 45 years old
- female > 55 year old, or has had hysterectomy, or is post menopausal
- smoker (or quit within past 6 months)
- BP > 140/90 mm Hg
- on BP medication
- blood cholesterol >200 mg/dL
- close blood relative who had heart attack/surgery at age <55 (male) or <65 (female)
- >20 pounds overweight (BMI > 30)
- pre-diabetes (see below for definition*) sedentary lifestyle (not exercising ≥ 30 min, 3×/week for past 3 months)
- **Negative risk factor:** high-serum HDL cholesterol ≥ 60 mg/dL (1.6 mmol/L)

TABLE 3.2 *(Continued)*

Other Risk Factors (RISK ± supervision):
• pregnancy
• musculoskeletal problems that limit physical activity
• client takes prescription medication that may influence exercise tolerance
• client has concerns about the safety of exercise

* ***Pre-diabetes:*** *Impaired Fasting Glucose (IFG) = fasting plasma glucose ≥ 100 mg/dL but < 126 mg/dL or Impaired Glucose Tolerance (IGT) = 2-hour values in oral glucose tolerance test (OGTT) ≥ 140 mg/dL but < 200 mg/dL confirmed by measurements on ≥ 2 separate occasions*

individual and program specific policies for preparticipation health screening and medical clearance, particularly for populations with known cardiovascular disease." (5)

Risk Algorithm: Assessing your Patient's Risk Level

If your patients answer *yes* to one or more of the questions on the PAR-Q, or trigger a referral based on their answers to the AHA/ACSM Screening Questionnaire (see Appendix), the clinician needs a means to effectively and efficiently assess these patients to stratify their risk level and determine the need for professional or clinical supervision with exercise, and whether preparticipation exercise testing is warranted.

While this book is addressed to all clinicians, this group of patients at potential risk for cardiovascular complications with exercise requires a more detailed assessment specifically by a physician. We similarly advise physicians not trained and comfortable with exercise testing to refer those patients in the *high risk* category, for whom they are not comfortable prescribing exercise, to consult cardiologists and exercise physiologists for further assessment.

The primary, though not the only, areas of focus for the assessment, are cardiovascular, pulmonary, or metabolic conditions. The Risk Stratification of Patients (Figure 3.3) outlines the assessment process, covering the areas of medical history (box 1), signs and symptoms (box 2), and risk factors (box 3). Questioning the patient about each of these symptoms or risk factors will determine his risk level. We will now review this process in detail.

Begin with the box: "Known CV, Pulmonary, Metabolic Disease?" The first box on page 38 (Table 3.2) details these conditions. If the patient has any of these conditions they fall into the HIGH RISK category. If not, then proceed to "Major Signs or Symptoms Suggestive of CV, Pulmonary, Metabolic Disease?" (See Table 3.2 for details.) Ask your patient if she experiences any of the symptoms listed in the box on Figure 3.3 and determine on examination if she has any of the signs listed. If yes, she falls into the HIGH RISK category and will require further assessment prior to beginning an exercise program.

If your patient does not present with a medical history or signs and symptoms of cardiovascular, pulmonary, or metabolic disease, proceed to box 3 to assess for cardiovascular disease risk factors. Ask your patient if he has any of the risk factors listed, and count the number of factors that apply to him. (See Table 3.2 for detailed list.) You should subtract one from the count of risk factors if the patient's HDL is >60 (a negative risk factor for cardiovascular disease). If the patient has less than two of these risk factors, he falls into the LOW RISK category (see below). If she has two or more of these risk factors, she is at MODERATE RISK (see below).

The final box in Table 3.2, "Other Risk Factors," will guide the patient toward using exercise modifications to address pregnancy, musculoskeletal problems, side effects of medications, or the patient's subjective concern about exercise. As will be described below, clinician discretion regarding the exercise prescription will likely be required to address these concerns. Chapter 13 details modifications recommended for special conditions.

In some cases, it may be difficult or impossible to ascertain the necessary information to accurately assess a patient's risk level. In such cases, clinicians are encouraged to use all available information and to make a conservative estimate of his or her patient's risk level. Note that this algorithm provides a guideline that may be modified at the discretion of the physician. Moreover, the patient's risk level may change over time. For example, if your patient's signs and symptoms (Fig. 3.3, Box 2) improve (*e.g.,* resolution of ischemic chest pain or shortness of breath with exertion), the patient may be advanced from HIGH RISK to MODERATE RISK. Similarly, if your patient's disease (Fig. 3.3, Box 1) is stable (*e.g.,* stable CVD, well controlled metabolic or pulmonary disease such as asthma, and other stable chronic diseases or conditions) she will remain at HIGH RISK; however, the intensity of her exercise may be increased at the discretion of her physician or after consultation with a cardiologist or other specialist. A patient in the moderate risk category based on cardiac risk factors may be progressed to LOW RISK if the risk factors resolve (*e.g.,* quitting smoking, losing weight, or no longer being sedentary).

The Risk Levels

Placement of your patient in the HIGH, MODERATE, or LOW RISK categories helps the physician determine the need for preparticipation screening and supervision during exercise. Please see Table 3.3 to determine the level of supervision and need for further screening based on the planned intensity of exercise for each of the risk categories.

If your patient answered *no* to all 7 questions on the PAR-Q, she is in the LOW RISK category. Such patients are generally safe to begin an exercise program without supervision or further medical clearance. Please refer to fol-

---

TABLE 3.3 Assessing Your Patient's Medical Risk
Associated with Exercise

Assessing your patient's medical risk:

- Ask your patient to fill out the simple PAR-Q. If she answers *no* to all questions, she is likely safe to begin exercising independently
- If she answers *yes* to any of the 7 questions, proceed to the attached algorithm and ask about the history, signs and symptoms, or risk factors in each of the three boxes to determine her risk level:
  - HIGH RISK: should undergo further medical testing before starting an exercise program
  - MODERATE RISK: Patient is safe to begin light- or moderate-intensity exercise (should undergo further medical assessment before partaking in vigorous-intensity exercise)
  - LOW RISK: Patient is safe to begin exercising without further assessment

---

lowing chapters on motivation and exercise progression to assist your patient in initiating an exercise program.

Patients who fall under the MODERATE RISK category are generally safe to begin low- or moderate-level exercise without further medical clearance. However, because these patients face an increased risk of an acute cardiovascular event, they should be referred for further medical assessment/clearance (including an exercise stress test) before initiating a *vigorous*-intensity exercise program. Patients placed in the MODERATE RISK category will require professional (non-medical) supervision, which is adequate to ensure safety while exercising (at a vigorous level) (11).

If the patient has been classified at the MODERATE RISK level because of cardiovascular, pulmonary, and/or metabolic risk factors, he should begin an exercise program under the supervision of a trained health professional (defined as "a health/fitness professional possessing a combination of academic training and certification equivalent to the ACSM Health/Fitness Instructor® or above" [11]). (See Chapter 2.)

If your patient presents with risk factors that are not cardiovascular, pulmonary, or metabolic in nature (*e.g.,* low-risk pregnancy), low- or moderate-intensity exercise can be initiated without supervision; however, certain modifications to the exercise program may be necessary. With these non-cardiovascular risk factors, you may need to use some discretion in determining whether vigorous-intensity exercise is safe for your patient, and whether she should begin her program under the supervision of a health or exercise professional. For example, if your patient has an isolated musculoskeletal injury to his wrist, this will not prevent him from exercising at any intensity, provided the exercise does not involve his wrist (walking or running, for example). This patient should be encouraged to exercise freely, choosing exercises that do not aggravate his wrist. Similarly, a patient who has concerns about the safety of exercise but has no other cardiovascular or metabolic risk factors, is safe to exercise at any intensity, but may benefit from beginning her program under the supervision of an exercise therapist or ACSM Certified Personal Trainer[SM].

Patients who fall under the HIGH RISK category are at risk for acute medical complications (primarily an acute cardiovascular event) and, therefore, require further medical assessment and clearance (including an exercise stress test) prior to beginning exercise. Unless you are specifically trained (and comfortable) conducting these tests, your patient should be referred to a qualified specialist. Patients in the high risk category will likely still be able to participate in a supervised exercise program, and should be encouraged to pursue the necessary tests in order to engage in an exercise program that is safe. High-risk patients, once cleared to begin a modified exercise program, will require clinical supervision from "a health/fitness professional possessing a combination of advanced college training and certification equivalent to the ACSM Registered Clinical Exercise Physiologist® and Exercise Specialist® or above" (11) who is aware of the patient's risk factors, as well as any modifications, precautions, and contraindication to the program.

Please see the section on cardiovascular disease in Chapter 13 for further discussion of exercise testing results and absolute and relative contraindications to exercise.

Levels of Supervision for Exercise

Once your patient's risk level has been determined, you will have a better sense of the intensity of the exercise in which she should participate. A second variable to consider is whether your patient will require supervision during his initial exercise sessions, and the level of training that the supervisor should have. Patients who fall into the low risk category do not require supervision for medical reasons. Those who are categorized as moderate risk may need supervision from someone with an ACSM Health/Fitness Instructor® (or equivalent) level of training. Use your professional discretion to decide if you feel that this is warranted, but initially take a conservative approach. Once patients in the high risk category have been cleared to begin a modified exercise program, they should do so under the clinical supervision of an ACSM Registered Clinical Exercise Physiologist® and Exercise Specialist®. This supervisor should be trained in basic life support, including CPR. Depending on the recommendations of the medical specialist, exercising in a facility with access to advanced cardiac life support may be necessary. Table 3.4 provides a summary of the exercise intensity restrictions and supervision recommendations for patients in each risk category.

TABLE 3.4 Summary of Exercise Considerations for Patients in Each Risk Category

	Low Risk	Moderate Risk	High Risk
Need further medical clearance before exercising at a **LOW** or **MODERATE** intensity?	No	No	Yes
Need further medical clearance before exercising at a **VIGOROUS** intensity?	No	Yes	Yes
Supervision required?	No	Often recommended—depends on the reason for falling into this category	Yes
Type of supervision recommended	None required	Professional*	Clinical**

* **Professional supervision** = under the supervision of a health/fitness professional possessing a combination of academic training and certification equivalent to the ACSM Health/Fitness Instructor® or above (11).

** **Clinical supervision** = under the direct supervision of a health/fitness professional possessing a combination of advanced college training and certification equivalent to the ACSM Registered Clinical Exercise Physiologist® and Exercise Specialist® or above (11).

There are situations in which your patients may want supervision for reasons other than a medical condition: if they need assistance in learning how to use weight machines at a fitness center; if they are particularly nervous about starting an exercise program; or if either you or your patient feels that exercising under supervision will provide the necessary motivation to continue regular exercise. Fitness center staff or private ACSM Certified Personal Trainers[SM] can assist with these needs.

CONCLUSION

In this chapter, we have begun the process of exercise prescription. We have outlined both the health risks that your patients face if they remain inactive, as well as the risks of exercising. Although most patients will benefit from participating in regular exercise, patients should be screened prior to initiating an exercise program. For many, this will consist of the short (7-question) PAR-Q, in which they are able to answer NO to each of the questions. These patients are safe to begin an exercise program of any intensity without supervision. For patients who answer YES to at least one of the PAR-Q questions, the screening process needs to continue to assess their level of risk. The risk level (low, moderate, or high) that your patient is assessed at will determine a) whether she needs further medical assessment prior to beginning an exercise program, b) the intensity at which she is safe to exercise, and c) whether she needs supervision during her physical activity.

This assessment of health "readiness" is the first of two exercise readiness assessments. In the next chapter, we will introduce you to the second component: "mental readiness."

References

1. Haskell WL, Lee IM, Pate RR, Powell KE, Blair SN, Franklin BA, Macera CA, Heath GW, Thompson PD, Bauman A. Physical activity and public health: updated recommendation from the American College of Sports Medicine and the American Heart Association. Med Sci Sports Exer 2007 Aug;39(8):1423–34.
2. Fletcher GF, Blair SN, Blumenthal J, Caspersen C, Chaitman B, Epstein S, Falls H, Froelicher ES, Froelicher VF, Pina IL. Statement on exercise: benefits and recommendations for physical activity programs for all Americans: a statement for health professionals by the Committee on Exercise and Cardiac Rehabilitation of the Council on Clinical Cardiology, American Heart Association. Circulation 1992 Jul;86(1):340–4.
3. Thompson PD, Buchner D, Pina IL, Balady GJ, Williams MA, Marcus BH, Berra K, Blair SN, Costa F, Franklin B, Fletcher GF, Gordon NF, Pate RR, Rodriguez BL, Yancey AK, Wenger NK; American Heart Association Council on Clinical Cardiology Subcommittee on Exercise, Rehabilitation, and Prevention; American Heart Association Council on Nutrition, Physical Activity, and Metabolism Subcommittee on Physical Activity. Exercise and physical activity in the prevention and treatment of atherosclerotic cardiovascular disease: A statement from the Council on Clinical Cardiology (Subcommittee on Exercise, Rehabilitation, and Prevention) and the Council on Nutrition, Physical Activity, and Metabolism (Subcommittee on Physical Activity). Circulation 2003 Jun 24;107(24):3109–16.
4. Department of Health and Human Services. Physical activity and health: a report of the Surgeon General. Atlanta, GA: USDHHS, Centers for Disease Control and Prevention; 1996, 300 p.
5. Doyle AJ. Preparticipation health screening and risk stratification. In: American College of Sports Medicine, editor. ACSM's guidelines for exercise testing and prescription. 8th ed. Philadelphia: Lippincott Williams & Wilkins. 2009.
6. American College of Sports Medicine Position Stand and American Heart Association. Recommendations for cardiovascular screening, staffing, and emergency policies at health/fitness facilities. Med Sci Sports Exerc 1998 Jun;30(6):1009–18.
7. Fletcher GF, Balady GJ, Amsterdam EA, Chaitman B, Eckel R, Fleg J, Froelicher VF, Leon AS, Piña IL, Rodney R, Simons-Morton DA, Williams MA, Bazzarre T. Exercise standards for testing and training: a statement for healthcare professionals from the American Heart Association. Circulation 2001 Oct 2;104(14):1694–740.
8. Maron BJ, Araujo CG, Thompson PD, Fletcher GF, de Luna AB, Fleg JL, Pelliccia A, Balady GJ, Furlanello F, Van Camp SP, Elosua R, Chaitman BR, Bazzarre TL;

World Heart Federation; International Federation of Sports Medicine; American Heart Association Committee on Exercise, Cardiac Rehabilitation, and Prevention. Recommendations for preparticipation screening and the assessment of cardiovascular disease in masters athletes: an advisory for healthcare professionals from the working groups of the World Heart Federation, the International Federation of Sports Medicine, and the American Heart Association Committee on Exercise, Cardiac Rehabilitation, and Prevention. Circulation 2001 Jan 16;103(2):327–34.

9. Maron BJ, Thompson PD, Puffer JC, McGrew CA, Strong WB, Douglas PS, Clark LT, Mitten MJ, Crawford MH, Atkins DL, Driscoll DJ, Epstein AE. Cardiovascular preparticipation screening of competitive athletes. A statement for health professionals from the Sudden Death Committee (clinical cardiology) and Congenital Cardiac Defects Committee (cardiovascular disease in the young), American Heart Association. Circulation 1996 Aug 15;94(4):850–6.

10. American Association of Cardiovascular and Pulmonary Rehabilitation. Guidelines for cardiac rehabilitation and secondary prevention programs. 4th ed. Champaign: Human Kinetics; 2004. 288 p.

11. Garber ME_. Exercise prescription. In: American College of Sports Medicine, editor. ACSM's guidelines for exercise testing and prescription. 8th ed. Philadelphia: Lippincott Williams & Wilkins. 2009, pp. 152–182.

APPENDIX: AHA/ACSM HEALTH/FITNESS FACILITY PREPARTICIPATION SCREENING QUESTIONNAIRE

Assess your health status by marking all true statements

HISTORY

You have had:

_____ a heart attack

_____ heart surgery

_____ cardiac catheterization coronary

_____ angioplasty (PTCA)

_____ pacemaker/implantable cardiac defibrillator

_____ rhythm disturbance

_____ heart valve disease

_____ heart failure

_____ heart transplantation

_____ congenital heart disease

Symptoms:

_____ You experience chest discomfort with exertion

_____ You experience unreasonable breathlessness

_____ You experience dizziness, fainting, or blackouts

_____ You take heart medications

Other health issues:

_____ You have diabetes

_____ You have asthma or other lung disease

_____ You have burning or cramping sensation in your lower legs when walking short distances

_____ You have musculoskeletal problems that limit your physical activity.

_____ You have concerns about the safety of exercise

_____ You take prescription medication(s)

_____ You are pregnant.

If you marked any of these statements in this section, consult your physician or other appropriate health care provider before engaging in exercise. You may need to use a facility with a medically qualified staff.

CARDIOVASCULAR RISK FACTORS

_____ You are a man older than 45 years.

_____ You are a woman older than 55 years, have had a hysterectomy, or are postmenopausal

_____ You smoke, or quit smoking within the previous 6 months.

_____ Your blood pressure is >140/90 mm Hg.

_____ You do not know your blood pressure.

_____ You take blood pressure medication.

_____ Your blood cholesterol level is >200 mg/dL.

_____ You do not know your cholesterol level.

_____ You have a close blood relative who had a heart attack or heart surgery before age 55 (father or brother) or age 65 (mother or sister).

_____ You are physically inactive (i.e., you get <30 minutes of physical activity on at least 3 days per week).

_____ You are >20 pounds overweight

If you marked two or more of the statements in this section you should consult your physician or other appropriate health care provider before engaging in exercise. You might benefit from using a facility with a professionally qualified exercise staff to guide your exercise program.

_____ None of the above

You should be able to exercise safely without consulting your physician or other appropriate health care provider in a self-guided program or almost any facility that meets your exercise program needs.

Modified from American College of Sports Medicine and American Heart Association. ACSM/AHA Joint Position Statement: Recommendations for cardiovascular screening, staffing, and emergency policies at health/fitness facilities. Medicine and Science in Sports and Exercise 1998;30:1009–18.

CHAPTER 4

Mobilizing Motivation: Basic Concepts

Steven Jonas

INTRODUCTION

As mentioned in the Introduction, the United States is awash in information about both *what* to do in exercise and *how* to do it. If those were the key factors in helping people to become regular exercisers, the country would be awash with regular exercisers, too. However, it has become quite obvious, as the U.S. population becomes heavier and less active, the "what" and "how," although important, are not the central factors in helping people to make health-promoting personal behavior changes. Over time it has become clear that it is the *motivation to make changes* and *how to go about mobilizing it* that are the central factors. No one is going to be able to make a health-promoting behavior change and then stick with it indefinitely if they are not properly motivated to become healthier and stay that way, have not mobilized their own motivation to do so, cannot maintain their motivation indefinitely, and cannot first gain control of the process and then stay in control of it.

THE NATURAL HISTORY OF HEALTHY BEHAVIOR CHANGE

If one is leading a sedentary lifestyle and is not engaging in job-related or leisure-time extraneous physical exertion, then becoming a regular exerciser will obviously mark a big change. However, can a person simply say, at any given time in life, "OK, I'm going to start a program now, I will stick with it indefinitely, and a lifetime pattern of regular exercise will be the result," and be assured of success?

First of all, each person's health status changes over time. It is a rare person who can be entirely healthy at any one time. A sound aphorism that applies to all health-promoting lifestyle or behavior changes is: "We can never be perfect; we can always get better." In the course of our own lifetimes, each of us will engage in some particular aspect of "getting better," such as becoming a regular exerciser; but *when* this happens varies widely from person to person. We will repeat this because it is an important premise of our whole approach: *Perfection is not the objective here; becoming healthier and thus hap-*

pier is. Different people change at different rates at different times in their lives. Different people achieve different goals at different times in their lives. But if they do make changes and change successfully, motivation and their ability to mobilize it are at the center of the effort. Therefore, we are going to spend a fair amount of time and space in this book discussing the subject.

MOTIVATION: BASIC CONCEPTS

Definition

Most people know in general terms what they are thinking about when they say, "I've got to get motivated," "My motivation is high for this one," or, alternatively, "Gee, I just can't seem to get motivated." But few of us can immediately put into words exactly what we mean when we use the term. Indeed, even among health professionals, many who use it frequently don't define it in so many words. However, for this discussion, it is helpful to have a written definition. Our definition is:

> "Motivation is *a state of mind* (characterized as an emotion, feeling, desire, idea, or intellectual understanding; or a psychological, physiological, or health need mediated by a mental process) which leads to the taking of one or more actions."

Or, briefly:

> "Motivation is mental process that connects a thought or a feeling with an action."

Thus, motivation is based in the mind. It is a thought or set of thoughts. It is not something tangible. In other than psychopathologically self-destructive persons, motivation is always potentially there, even if inactive, for it is essential to self-preservation and the underlying human striving to be healthy. Thus, "getting motivated" is not a question of developing or importing the mind-state. It is rather a matter of *activating a presently quiescent process,* of *mobilizing it,* of *removing barriers to its expression.* If a patient is having a hard time "getting motivated" but seems ready to start (see the Stages of Change, which follows), the clinician's task is to help the patient locate these barriers and then help him or her to mobilize the mental process needed to remove them.

Among the common barriers to effective motivation mobilization are: "I really don't want to do this"; "I know I'll just never be able to get started"; "I just know I don't have the time"; "One day I want to and the next day I don't"; and fear of failure once one does get started, that "I-know-that-I-just-won't-be-able-to-do-it" feeling. Throughout the rest of this chapter, you will find suggestions for helping patients work through these types of internal obstacles to mobilizing motivation. Central to doing that is considering the question, "What patient needs are being met, what function is being served by the patient's *not* exercising on a regular basis?" As one wag once put it, "Are your risk factors in such tip-top shape that you can get through life staying healthy, *without* exercising?"

Motivation: Mental Process and Action

When we talk about either "being motivated" or "lacking motivation," we are referring to various states of mind that will either impel us to undertake an action or hinder us from doing so. There are three phases in "finding" or "developing" motivation: first, *experiencing* an emotional and/or intellectual thought processes of the motivational type; second, establishing a clear mental pathway between those thoughts and the *potential* for taking the related action; and third, *taking the action* as the result of being motivated.

EFFECTIVE MOTIVATION ALMOST ALWAYS COMES FROM WITHIN

The scientific literature is clear that in most cases, to be effective, motivation must be inner-directed, *e.g.,* "I want to do this for me, to look better, feel better, feel better about myself, for me, not for anyone else" (1). External motivation— "I'm doing this for my spouse (or significant other or friend or children/parents or employer/co-workers)"—almost invariably leads to feelings of guilt, anxiety, anger, and frustration and then, often, to injury and/or quitting. If your patient wants to look better, feel better, be fitter, and feel better about himself or herself, *for himself or herself,* for no one else, then he has *inner* motivation. If the patient views simply as an extra benefit whatever good the changes do for her in others' eyes, then she has inner motivation.

With inner motivation your patient will be able to take control of the way he exercises and eats (and smokes or not, and drinks out-of-control or not, etc.). With inner motivation, the chances are excellent that he will become a regular exerciser, slowly, gradually, and carefully. The one exception to the inner-directed rule is when the person can honestly say, "I'm doing this for someone else because it will make *me* feel good and feel good about *myself* if I make them happy." However, even in this case, the motivation is still coming from inside. Because no one can effectively motivate anyone else, you must be able to clearly see your role as a clinician, with its natural limits.

You can guide your patient through the processes of internal motivation-mobilization and goal-setting leading to self-discovery and action, provide positive reinforcement, model the role, offer technical assistance—but that's all. You cannot motivate other people for lifestyle behavior change. You can only help patients locate their own motivation and mobilize it within themselves by taking control of the process.

TAKING CONTROL

Taking control is a critical concept to stress in the process of helping patients to locate/unblock/mobilize motivation. Indeed, it is the fifth and final step in the wellness motivation mobilization pathway described in detail in Chapter 5. When your patient takes control, she is deciding what she wants to do with his or her body; she is deciding to engage in physical activity regularly, perhaps to do some things, let's say in a sport, that she has never done, or ever contemplated doing.

Taking control is central to both starting a regular exercise program and sticking with it. And there is much to take control of: whether to undertake a change process at all; what goals to set; which sport(s) and/or activity(s) to engage in. Making choices, of course, as we said in the Introduction to this book, means taking responsibility oneself, for oneself. Taking control and taking responsibility are both mental processes known to psychologists to be powerful motivational tools.

THE PROCESS OF CHANGE: PSYCHOLOGICAL CONSIDERATIONS

The Stages of Change

In helping patients to mobilize their motivation and then engage in behavioral change, it is important for both of you to understand that, in most people, such change does not occur overnight. In fact, programs that focus solely on the behaviors without attending to the motivational process that underlies behavioral change, are more likely than not to fail.

A psychological model of the gradual process that underlies the mobilization of motivation for change, originally developed by Prochaska and DiClemente (2) and updated in the 1990s (3–6), is widely used. (There are others that are valid, too. We are simply most comfortable with this one.) This description and analysis of the change process is helpful in understanding how and why motivation is successfully mobilized, as well as in understanding the factors that lead to failure to do so. In their revision of the original model, Prochaska, DiClemente, and Norcross identify what they call "The Six Stages of Change": precontemplation, contemplation, preparation, action, maintenance, and termination. As Prochaska pointed out in terms that are still valid, "In this stage approach to change, taking direct action to change one's behavior is only one of six stages. What people do in the stages preceding action and what they do in the stages following action are at least as important as the action they take" (4).

And so, the stages (see the summary at the end of this section, in Three-Minute Drill 4-1):

THREE-MINUTE DRILL, 4 – 1

The Six Stages of Change

1. Precontemplation	5. Maintenance
2. Contemplation	a. Lapse
3. Preparation/Planning	b. Relapse
4. Action	6. Termination (Permanent Maintenance)

PRECONTEMPLATION

The person has not yet decided or determined that he has a problem that requires a solution, taking action, and making a change. Therefore, he or she does not intend to take any action within the upcoming six months. He may be unaware, or not fully aware, of the true benefits of making change or may be demoralized from past unsuccessful attempts at change. Thus, he accepts his present state of being, either happily or unhappily.

CONTEMPLATION

In this stage, the person starts to become more aware of herself. She recognizes that she is engaging in a behavior, such as sedentary lifestyle, that actually constitutes a problem. She begins to look at different aspects of change and to assess just how this current behavior is affecting her. In this stage, she seriously intends to take action within the next six months or so but is not prepared to do it just yet. She is well aware of the advantages of making change, and at least part of her mind is in favor of doing it. But, at the same time, she is still concerned about the cons of change-making (that is, she is ambivalent—see the next paragraph), and may be convinced that success will be hard, if not impossible, to achieve.

As Miller and Rollnick have put it, "Once some awareness of the problem arises, the person enters a period characterized by *ambivalence:* the 'contemplation' stage. The contemplator both considers change and rejects it" (7, emphasis added). Some people can remain in the contemplation stage for quite some time, even though upon originally entering it they fully intended to make a change within six months. Those who will proceed to the next stage are able to begin seeing themselves in the future as persons who behave differently than they do at present.

PREPARATION/PLANNING

In this stage, the person is seriously planning to engage in behavior change within the next month or so. Upon entering this stage, the person has, in the common parlance, "become motivated." One has found those thoughts that will activate him, that will overcome his or her ambivalent feelings and his doubts that he can, in fact, succeed. He consciously chooses to engage in a new set of behaviors and believes that positive change will indeed be possible.

ACTION

The next step of the change process is taking the action itself. But let us reiterate that you will not be doing the best job for your patients if you just focus on the action, regular exercise using one or more sports or activities, and the details of workout schedules and so forth. Those elements are important, of course; but you will be doing the best job if you are aware of the whole motivational process. You will be doing your best job if you are able to identify in which of the Stages of Change each of your patients is at the time of the visit. You will be doing your best job if you help patients recognize when they have mobilized their motivation (see Chapters 5 and 6) and are truly ready to take an action with an excellent chance that they will succeed.

MAINTENANCE

This is the step that all people who have commenced an action want to reach. Once they have become regular exercisers, they want to remain one, indefinitely. There are three different possible departures from the Maintenance stage: Lapse, Relapse, and Termination. (For regular exercise, we refer to "Termination" as "Permanent Maintenance"; see Termination (Permanent Maintenance), which follows).

Lapse   Lapse is a temporary abandonment of the positive behavior, followed by a quick return to it. Lapse does not produce any significant alteration in progress towards established goals or, having achieved them, any significant modification in fitness or body configuration. Lapse is fine, can be fun for a limited time, and is perfectly normal. Worrisome is what is called relapse.

Relapse   Relapse is abandonment of the positive behavior that has produced the desired outcome, to the extent that the outcome disappears. The program of regular exercise is given up indefinitely, the good feelings, changes in body shape, and increased strength and endurance gained from doing it vanish. To reverse relapse requires first figuring out what happened, why the relapse occurred. Then, it requires going back to the planning, or possibly even the contemplation stage, re-commencing the change process and re-mobilizing motivation.

In dealing with relapse, it is important to understand that just as being sedentary is not a sign of moral failure or weakness, neither is relapsing. It just means that one wasn't really ready the first time around, that one was not effectively motivated, and/or perhaps that the goals set were unrealistic. If your patient experiences relapse, it is important that she does not let the natural disappointment turn into discouragement or demoralization. There are often good reasons for the occurrence. It happens to many people and does not necessarily mean that they will not eventually achieve Termination or Permanent Maintenance.

TERMINATION (PERMANENT MAINTENANCE)

As used by Prochaska and associates, *Termination* means that your patient has gone beyond relapse. They use this word to describe this stage because most of the behavior changes they are talking about entail permanently *stopping* some *negative* behavior, such as cigarette smoking or eating a high-fat diet, rather than incorporating a positive one into one's life and then staying with it. With regular exercise, we are, of course, talking about doing something *positive,* rather than not doing something negative, indefinitely. Thus, for the behavior regular exercise, *Permanent Maintenance* is a more appropriate term.

Lapse may still occur and, as we will see in Chapter 10, is good periodically for the regular exerciser. The pauses should not last too long, however, because the person may experience significant muscular pain when returning to the activity. But a lapse can show your patient that to stay in control over the long run, one doesn't have to be perfect.

It happens that for many, once the permanent maintenance stage is reached for the first time, regular exercise is a self-reinforcing, positive behavior. That is because most regular exercisers find that if they stop for too long, they just do not feel well and are almost impelled to take up their activity(s) again. There are, in fact, some regular exercisers who, because of this phenomenon, find it difficult to take the occasional pause-for-recharging break that is beneficial for most.

The PACE Project (8) has simplified the Stages of Change to a triage system that allows the clinician to tailor the message to the patients according to their readiness for change. In short, the Precontemplative patients are informed about the benefits of exercise in an effort to move them toward at least contemplative regular physical activity. Patients at the other end of the spectrum—in the Action through the Permanent Maintenance phases—and who are already regularly active are counseled to maintain or possibly increase their exercise and are taught about injury prevention, rotation of exercise, and other subjects that are covered in Chapter 9. The middle group—of contemplative and planning patients who are not yet active—require counseling and exercise prescription to initiate their physical activity programs. Please see Figure 4.1 for questions to determine which stage of change your patient is at regarding physical activity.

Ambivalence

Ambivalence is a state of mind characterized by coexisting but conflicting feelings about a contemplated action, another person, or a situation in which one

Physical Activity States of change

Instructions: For each question below, please fill in the square Yes or No. Please be sure to follow the instructions carefully.

Yes   No

1. I am currently physically active.   ☐Y ☐N

2. I intend to become more physically active in the next 6 months. ☐Y ☐N

For activity to be regular, it must add up to a total of 30 or more minutes per day and be done at least 5 days per week. For example, you could take one 30-minute walk or three 10-minute walks each day.

Yes   No

3. I currently engage in regular physical activity.   ☐Y ☐N

4. I have been regularly physically active for the past 6 months.   ☐Y ☐N

	ITEM			
Stage	1	2	3	4
Precontemplation	No	No	—	—
Contemplation	No	Yes	—	—
Preparation	Yes	—	No	—
Action	Yes	—	Yes	No
Maintenance	Yes	—	Yes	Yes

Figure 4.1 • Physical Activity: Stages of Change

finds oneself (7). Feeling ambivalent about making a behavior change is perfectly normal. Virtually everyone who even thinks about making a behavior change experiences it. Allowing ambivalence to paralyze decision-making, however, is a problem. Handled correctly, the process of resolving ambivalent feelings can help your patient get started on the road to success in regular exercise. A key to success in dealing with ambivalence is to accept that it will always be present to some extent. Sometimes the ambivalent feelings will be weaker, sometimes stronger. It is what one does in response to the feelings that determines their impact, of course.

From the literature on the addictive behaviors, Miller and Rollnick note (7, p. ix):

> It is a common problem for people to seem 'stuck,' to persist in patterns of behavior that clearly harm them and those around them. It is an old complaint: 'I do not understand my own actions. For I do not do what I want, but I do the very thing I hate' (Romans 7:15, Revised Standard Version).

This is a behavior pattern familiar to many health professionals who have tried to help persons with unresolved ambivalence, or an ambivalence which these persons are not able to resolve in a positive direction.

Wherever your patient is in the change process, even when he has achieved his or her goals, he needs to be reminded occasionally that ambivalent feelings are perfectly normal. It is how these feelings are handled, how they are responded to that determines whether they will trip one up or not get in one's way. If ambivalence *destroys* commitment, that is a problem. If it simply *questions* commitment, if it does nothing more than take your patient on a temporary detour, it can lead to a strengthening of resolve to proceed forward.

An important aspect of helping your patient to mobilize his or her motivation, thereby sending, her successfully on his or her way through the six stages, is helping her to effectively deal with ambivalence. Again, fighting the existence of the feelings does not work, in most cases. The person who is stuck with unresolved feelings of ambivalence is a person who, in many cases, must look beyond or behind those feelings to determine why she has them in the first place. Some people can do this on their own; others need help. Usually, however, dealing with ambivalent feelings about becoming a regular exerciser is a lot easier than, for instance, dealing with ambivalent feelings about another person or one's job, and should not require external intervention beyond what the non-psychotherapist health professional can offer.

Before starting the new behavior, your patient will have to be able to get enough onto the, "Yes, I would like to change, yes I can change" track to indeed do so. She does not have to completely resolve her ambivalence to do so. The "I can do this" feelings will simply have to outweigh the "I can't do this" feelings, not necessarily totally obliterate them.

Dealing With the Need for Immediate Gratification

In contemporary American society, immediate gratification and the promise of it are common elements of our social consciousness. Urgings to indulge in immediate gratification come at us in many forms and from many directions. For example, we have been told, if you have a sudden hunger for that certain burger, you had better go right out and satisfy that hunger, right now. And you are told to do that regardless of what else is going on in your life at the time. Then there are the instant scratch-off games in various public and private lotteries. No need to wait. You will know right away if you are a winner.

Our consumer-oriented economy is built on immediate gratification? "You do want this new car, new TV, new camcorder, new fancy cell-phone, right now, don't you? Don't have the money? Not to worry. Don't even think about waiting until you have saved up for it. Just borrow it." So, too, is one promised immediate gratification by those "14-Day Wonder Diets" (none of which work for weight maintenance over the long-run, of course).

In a society that promotes immediate gratification, how does one deal with this problem? Well, it may be possible to deal with it cognitively, by helping your patient to understand where the drive for immediate gratification comes from and that it can only harm, not help. But in addition to, or in place of, that approach, there is a kind of immediate gratification that can be obtained in the process of taking control itself. It won't hurt and will help, very much so. It's a *mental* immediate gratification, not a physically measured one like scale weight. It is the immediate gratification that comes from taking control, taking responsibility, realizing self-empowerment realizing self-efficacy, and doing something new and different. Yes, mobilizing motivation can itself lead to feelings of immediate gratification.

In less than a month of regularly exercising, simply with ordinary walking 10–20 minutes three times a week (see Chapter 7), without any significant physical changes yet apparent, your patient may well start to think: "Wow, I can really do this. I can really free up some time for myself, get a pair of walking shoes on, go outside, and do it. I can take control and make a positive change in my life, right now, and that feels good." That's immediate gratification of the positive kind.

Guilt Feelings as a Motivator

When contemplating a positive lifestyle behavior change, some people have such thoughts as, "I *have* to," "I *ought* to," and "I *should*" (in contrast with "I want to" and "I would like to"). "Have to," "ought to," and "should" are all representations of feeling guilty, that is, "a painful feeling of self-reproach resulting from a belief that one has done something wrong or immoral" (9). Experience has shown that as a motivator, guilt feelings, whether coming from inside or induced by others, do not work very well (7, pp. 5–7). They elicit what the psychologists call "resistance" and/or "denial."

The guilt-inducing "you-gotta" approach, whether self- or other-inflicted, is generally counter-productive. In lay language, "resistance" and "denial" translate as "I don't wanna" and "Problem? What problem?" Feeling guilty about anything eventually also leads to frustration and, then, anger. Because we do not like feeling either angry or frustrated, the presence of those thoughts is likely to lead us to quit doing what we are doing. In summary, guilt feelings almost invariably lead to frustration, anger, and then to quitting. Not a good motivator.

MOBILIZING MOTIVATION FOR REGULAR EXERCISE: THREE CENTRAL THOUGHTS TO KEEP IN MIND

Getting Started: "It's the Regular, Not the Exercise"

It is important for both you and your patients to recognize that the first challenge of becoming a regular exerciser for most people is the **regular,** not the **exercise.** Most people are aware that they "should exercise," that it is "good for them," even that they will "feel better," if they do. But for many people with a busy, full life, the schedule and other time demands just do not provide room for exercise on a regular basis. Indeed, for most people, the hard part of regular exercise is the regular, not the exercise.

The correct first step for many is to learn not a particular sport or activity but learn that they can indeed make or find the time, if they are motivated to do so. And that by behaviorally going about making the time first, as suggested by the modest beginning training programs that are set out in Chapters 7–10, they can reinforce their motivation. Thus, the focus of the first 2 to 4 weeks of an exercise program should be on the matter of "finding the time/making the time," most often using ordinary walking as the exercise, rather than on one or more exercises/activities/sports that might become part of one's life. In recommending this approach, you will both deal with the patient's reality and show him that you understand that reality.

Gradual Change

"Gradual change leads to permanent changes" is another helpful guiding concept for the person who is becoming a regular exerciser. Thus, as you will see in the Starting from Scratch program in Chapter 10, it is highly recommended that a previously sedentary person start just with ordinary walking for 10 minutes or so, three times a week. After a couple of weeks, she can increase the time spent, and perhaps the frequency; and after a couple more weeks, perhaps the speed.

The hardier, more energetic, and perhaps more motivated soul may move through this regimen more quickly. However, all should be counseled against going out for an hour, at full tilt, on that first day, or even on the fifth or tenth. For most people, "too much, too soon" is bound to lead to muscle pain, perhaps to injury, and an greater likelihood of quitting early. A *gradual* increase in time spent, distance covered, and speed is the proven formula for sticking with it.

Goal-Setting

Finally, the key to the whole thing, to mobilizing motivation and to keep it going, is goal-setting. It is the central element in the five-step process known as the Wellness Motivational Pathway for Healthy Living (which we will get to in the next chapter). The exercise prescription most usefully negotiated with the patient provides both Specific, Measurable, Achievable, Realistic, and Timely (SMART) goals for the patient to pursue, and a SMART pathway for reaching them. It is what makes all efforts at behavior change work. We will cover it in detail in the next chapter. In the meantime, you will find two 3-minute drills, Three-Minute Drills 4-2 and 4-3, that can help you and your patients to focus on these subjects.

CONCLUSION

Mobilizing Motivation is the central issue in making any health-promoting behavior change, as we have said before and will say again. It is also the hardest part. That is why we spend so much time on the subject in this book. In

---

THREE-MINUTE DRILL, 4 – 2

The Central Concepts of Successful Behavior Change

1. There *are* defined stages of change.
2. Everyone is subject to ambivalence.
3. Gradual change leads to permanent changes.
4. Setting goals and writing them down are key.
5. The need for immediate gratification needs to be dealt with.
6. Guilt feelings are not effective as motivators.

THREE-MINUTE DRILL, 4 – 3

The Five Elements of SMART Goals

1. **S**pecific
2. **M**easurable
3. **A**chievable
4. **R**ealistic
5. **T**imely

---

this chapter we have laid the groundwork for understanding the mental processes involved and how we can help our patients understand these processes and make them work for each of our patients. In the next chapter we will see how they apply to the first of the two pathways to the mobilization of motivation that we provide for you in this book. We should note that this approach to getting started as a regular exerciser has been summarized in another ACSM publication that you may find helpful for your patients (10).

References

1. Curry SJ, Wagner EH, Grothaus LC. Evaluation of intrinsic and extrinsic motivation interventions with a self-help smoking cessation program. J Consult Clin Psychol. 1991 April;59(2): 318.
2. Prochaska JO, DiClemente CC. Transtheoretical therapy: toward a more integrative model of change. Psychotherapy: Theory, Research, and Practice. 1982 Fall;19(3): 276–88.
3. Prochaska JO, DiClemente CC, Norcross JC. In search of how people change: applications to addictive behavior. Am Psychol 1992 Jan;47(1):102–110.
4. Prochaska JO. Working in harmony with how people change naturally. The Weight Control Digest. 1993 Fall;3(3):249.
5. Prochaska JO, Velicer WF, Rossi JF, Goldstein MG, Marcus BH, Rakowski W, Fiore C. Stages of change and decisional balance in 12 problem behaviors. Health Psychol. 1994 Jan;13(1):39–46.
6. Prochaska JO, Velicer WF. The transtheoretical model of behavior change. Am J Health Promot. 1997 Sept/Oct;12(1):38–48.

7. Miller WR, Rollnick S. Motivational interviewing: preparing people to change addictive behavior. New York: The Guilford Press; 1991. 348 p. A more recent edition of this work, under the title Motivational interviewing: preparing people for change, was published by Guilford in 2002.

8. Center for Health Interventions and Technology, LLC (US). PACE: patient-centered assessment and counseling for exercise and nutrition. San Diego (CA): San Diego Center for Health Interventions; 1999. 112 p.

9. Webster's new world dictionary. 2nd college ed. New York: The World Publishing Co.; 1970.

10. Jonas S. Getting ready to exercise. In: American College of Sports Medicine (US). ACSM fitness book. Champaign (IL): Human Kinetics; 2003. p. 41–58.

CHAPTER 5

Mobilizing Motivation: The Wellness Pathway

Steven Jonas

INTRODUCTION

As noted, in our view there is no single approach to helping patients become regular exercisers that will work for everyone. Therefore, in this book, we present you with two different approaches to doing so. There are others, to be sure, but these are the two with which we have had experience and for which we have evidence of success, at least in practice. In this chapter we cover "The Wellness Motivational Pathway (WMP)" approach. In the next chapter we cover the approach that is known as "Climbing Mount Lasting Change." Each will be helpful for different clinicians helping different patients with the practicalities of becoming regular exercisers, once they have mobilized their motivation through one pathway or the other. These are covered in Chapters 7, 8, 9, and 10.

As noted in Chapter 4, we talk about *mobilizing* motivation, not "developing" it or "acquiring" it. Your patient will not "get" motivation from the outside, or "find" it upon looking under the pillow, opening a bottle of pills, (even the so-called exercise pill) or even talking with you. It happens that most otherwise healthy people are inherently motivated to be, become, and remain healthy, because, as Thomas Jefferson said (see Introduction, p. 12) being healthy is a central part of living. As we have also noted, motivation is a process, not a thing or an endpoint. It is a process that links a thought, feeling, or emotion to an action. When people are "unmotivated," it does not mean that they lack the "right stuff." It simply means that the motivational process for the desired change has not been mobilized.

The most important commonality of the two approaches to mobilizing motivation that we present in this book is that each recognizes that the complexity of the motivational process can be broken down into a series of modifiable steps, at any of which you may intervene. Each has a series of steps for your patients to follow, fewer in the WMP, a larger number with smaller intervals between them in the behavior change pyramid. Different strokes for different folks, the comprehension of which principle by both you and your patients is key to helping people change their behaviors in positive ways.

Each approach to mobilizing motivation should be seen as the framework for establishing a continuous mental feedback loop to be engaged in by your patients over time. The mental tasks are connected with one another and with the ongoing process of behavior change in a continuous, self-reinforcing, feedback loop. Each should also be seen as prescribing a pattern of thinking that will likely work for just about any health-promoting behavior change that a patient might undertake. While neither approach should be regarded as establishing a lock-step progression for a patient to follow, each does set up a pathway that is logical in its progression and which most people who use one or the other do follow, at least the first time through.

THE WELLNESS MOTIVATIONAL PATHWAY FOR HEALTHY LIVING

Recalling the Stages of Change discussed in Chapter 4 (1–3), the WMP provides your patient with the details of the bridge they need to cross in order to advance from the Planning Stage (III) to the Action Stage (IV). The WMP has been developed over time from observation, anecdotal interviews, and experience. While it has not been tested experimentally, as the behavior change pyramid has been, it appears to be a logical approach to how to cross the bridge from Stage III to Stage IV, and also appears to have no potential negative side-effects. It is the application of the classical program-planning model (4) to getting on to and staying on the wellness pathway, for life. The WMP is summarized in Three-Minute Drill 5-1.

The *WMP* has five steps:

1. The first step is *assessment,* both self and professional (for the latter, see Chapter 3). This first step is also essential to the behavior change pyramid.
2. The second step is *defining success,* for the person, by the person (with your help). To be effective for each individual, "success" has to be defined within his or her specific context, has to be realistic for him or her, and its achievement has to be within the realm of possibility for him or her.
3. The third step is *goal-setting.* This is the central element of the Wellness Motivational Pathway.

THREE-MINUTE DRILL, 5 – 1

The Five Steps of the Wellness Motivational Process for Healthy Living

1. Assessment (self and professional)
2. Defining success
3. Goal-setting
4. Establishing priorities
5. Taking control

4. The fourth is *establishing priorities* among the various sectors of a person's life. This is particularly important for achieving success if the person decides to become a regular exerciser by engaging in a planned leisure-time activity or sport.

5. The fifth is *taking control* of the whole process. This final step itself has eight elements (see Step 5—Taking Control, p. 67).

Everyone of us trying to change a health-related behavior has to begin somewhere. However, no exercise program or any other attempt at changing personal behavior, such as, for example, how you run your clinical practice, will work if you just jump right in with no goals, no plan, and no idea of where you are and how far you need or want to go. As you go through the process, it is helpful for both you and your patients to write down the elements of assessment, defining success, goal-setting, and establishing priorities, as you both proceed through each step. *Writing down thoughts focuses the mind for both you and your patients.* Now we shall turn to a consideration of the WMP in some detail.

Step 1—Assessment

Assessment has two components, assessment by oneself and assessment by others, usually health professionals. *Self*-assessment, as we shall see, is closely connected to goal-setting. Self-assessment, our focus here, is your patient asking himself herself questions such as:

- Where am I now in my life? How did I get here?
- What do I like about myself, my body? What do I not like?
- What is it about my body and mind that I am unhappy with that could be positively affected by exercising regularly?
- What would I like to change, if anything, and why?
- What is going on in my life that would facilitate behavior change? Inhibit it?
- Where am I now in my physical activity level?
- Have I tried regular exercise before and failed to stick with it?
- Currently, what do I estimate my potential to stick with an exercise program to be? (Realism is important here.)
- What unmet personal needs am I thinking about attempting to meet?
- Am I ready, really ready, to try it? Would I really like to change, even if it means giving up something I am accustomed to?
- Do I think that I can mobilize the mental strength (and it does take mental strength—there are no magic bullets to significantly change a personal behavior) if that is what I want or need to do?
- What has my previous experience with personal health behavior change been? Good? Bad? Some success? None? Will that help me this time around?
- What can I learn from experience that will help this time? Am I being realistic about this?
- Where am I in the Stages of Change?

An important element of self-assessment is looking at what one does well—for example, is the overweight person a non-smoker—as well as what one would like to do better. This element is especially significant in dealing with overweight, for example, on which our society tends to have a unitary focus to the exclusion of other factors in healthy living. Such a unitary, exclusionary focus can have a very negative influence on patients (5).

Thus, as your patient asks himself the questions above, he should also be thinking about:

- What is my self-image?
- Do I think of myself as good-looking? Attractive? Not attractive? Healthy? Unhealthy?
- What do I see when I look in the mirror?
- What kinds of feelings do those images elicit?
- And when I see, for instance, "fat," do others say that is a true reflection of reality?
- If I am planning to exercise to help in weight loss or simply to shape up a currently out-of-shape body, will I be able to use the facts that smaller-size clothing now fits and that my waist is getting smaller (that's at least smaller, if not small) as measures of success, rather than scale weight (which might or might not change much, even as I am redistributing body mass)?
- And further, if I am going to exercise primarily for weight loss, is my true goal to become really "thin," rather than somewhat thinner? Am I in reality looking for the "perfect body," something very few can achieve, even if there is such a thing? And if so, why?

Answering these questions is important in helping to define your patient's long-term goals and in mobilizing his or her motivation to achieve them.

Step 2—Defining Success for Oneself

How you approach the subject of success can be either helpful or rather harmful to your patients and to the process of setting and achieving their goals. Whether it concerns how to stop smoking, lose weight, or become a regular exerciser, just how your patient defines success for herself will have a major impact on the outcome. To be helpful and facilitating for health-promoting behavior change, success must be defined in terms that make sense for each patient and must be realistically achievable for him or her. If success is defined in terms that are objectively either impossible or difficult to achieve, then striving to achieve it becomes frustrating, inhibiting, and anger-provoking, and will eventually lead to quitting.

Thus, for your patients, the concept of "success" should be facilitating, not inhibiting. Also, it must be defined in terms of what they might reasonably achieve, for themselves, not for anyone else. Success, to put it yet another way, must be defined for each person in terms that make sense, that are realistic, for each person. For example, if someone is naturally slow of foot but decides to take up running, success should not be defined in terms of absolute speed, *e.g.,* "I will consider myself successful when I can run a mile in eight minutes." Success in this person's case might be better defined in terms of endurance, *e.g.,* "As my first objective, I want to be able to run for 20 minutes without stopping, at a comfortable pace." Once that objective is achieved, another can be set—if the person wishes to do so; for success must also be defined with the recognition that its meaning for any one person can change over time. In fact, for most people who experience success in regular exercise, it *will* change over time. However, at the beginning of the process, there is no way of knowing just how far an individual will get.

Finally, "endowment" (genetic potential) and "enhancement" (what one can do with it) must be considered. Whatever the proportion is between endowment and enhancement as the factors determining the achievement of success, very few people have the genetic potential for developing the body of a world class body builder (even if they were to use steroids), and very few have the potential of looking like a glamorous movie star (even with the assistance of plastic surgery). Nor do many people have it physically within themselves to run a marathon in under three hours. In setting goals for exercise, the role genes play in determining just what can be done must be recognized.

Consider: A strong genetic component is involved in the determination of body shape and size, potential strength, ability to increase muscle bulk by weightlifting, and achieving speed in any sport. At the same time, it can be emphasized that within one's genetic limitations significant changes in physical fitness, strength, speed to some extent, and certainly sports and athletics skills, can be made. Thus, goals can be, and in many cases should be, changed over time, but this should be done gradually and realistically. Although it is important for you to help your patients recognize their physical/genetic limitations, it is also important for you to help your patients explore their limits. What are they, really? For many persons who are not presently physically active, those limits are far wider than they ever imagined, especially if, as our patients explore them, they recognize their limitations as well. This is a subject to which we shall return in Chapters 12 and 15.

Step 3—Goal-Setting

Goal-setting is the central element of the WMP. We consider this to be the single most important undertaking in developing a successful program of regular exercise. What is it that I want to do and why do I want to do it? To where do I want to get? Why do I want to get there? For whom would I be making the change—others, or myself? What do I expect to get out of the change should I achieve it? What do I think I can reasonably expect to accomplish? Do I want to reduce my future risk for acquiring various diseases and negative health conditions? What do I hope to feel and be when I have made the contemplated changes in my life? What are the "give-ups," and can I, do I want to, commit to them? Arriving at satisfactory answers to these questions for oneself is absolutely key. Doing so provides the focus and the concentration one must have to have the best chance of success in the chosen endeavor. The initial goals set must be reasonable at the time they are set. Recognizing that what is considered to be realistic is likely to change over time, nothing can kill a change process faster than the setting of unrealistic, unachievable goals. As we have said previously, the goals set should be SMART, that is, Specific, Measurable, Achievable, Realistic, and Timely.

Once goals are established—goals that are reasonable for the person, that fit with his life and lifestyle and apparent natural abilities and inclinations—everything else, from planning a workout schedule, to buying a pair of walking shoes or a bicycle, to implementing the plan on a regular basis, is commentary. For the establishment of goals creates the mindset, the mental environment, which will permit and then facilitate what for most people is a major change in the way they live. It is the thinking that gets one going and keeps one going, whether in purposefully walking for 30 minutes five times per week, or using the stairs instead of the elevator and getting off the bus ten blocks from work everyday, or training for six months to run a marathon or an Olympic-distance triathlon.

Step 4—Establishing Priorities

Establishing priorities among the various possible health-promoting behaviors and between the planned personal health-promotion program and the rest of one's life is the next step. Creating balance among the set of behavior-change goals, and between the new goals and the rest of one's life is central to making the whole process work. If the person has set more than one goal, what is their ranking? Which is considered to be the most important to achieve? Which the least? In addition, what about priorities between the new goal(s) (in the case of athletics and other leisure-time activities) and other important things that are going on in other parts of the patient's life, like relationships with family and friends, and employment? If juggling needs to be done, it will be very helpful to do some thinking about that and, yes, set priorities.

Making the Time. As we have noted at the beginning of this chapter, becoming a regular exerciser intrudes on one's time for the rest of one's life. This aspect of the enterprise should not be swept under the rug. It needs to be examined carefully. How is time being spent now? Can your patient give up four hours of television a week? Can your patient get up 45 minutes earlier four days a week (including the two weekend days) and cut down on dawdling time by 15 minutes on each of those days? Can their spouse, for example, do some of the food shopping and cooking and help with some household chores? Spousal support is a very important element, not only in helping to make the time, but in helping to make the whole WMP work. If necessary, can she find some time during her workday to squeeze in time for working out? Better yet, can she take advantage of a health promotion program that many employers now sponsor, or can she make a suggestion to start one if it is not currently offered at her workplace?

Step 5—Taking Control

There are eight elements in *Taking Control* of the behavior that following through on the

Wellness Motivational Process is intended to lead to (Three-Minute Drill 5-2). Taking control of your life means "running your life instead of letting it run you." It is self-explanatory, but a difficult challenge for many of us to meet. We have already considered most of the elements in some detail; just a couple of additional points here.

"Exploring your limits while recognizing your limitations," as we have noted, means injecting realism into your program: playing to your strengths while at the same time dealing with your weaknesses realistically. Once having embarked on the journey of regular exercise, the traveler can be taken to places in his or her mind and with his or her body that he never previously dreamed of. The couch potato can become a marathoner, but one for whom the ultimate achievement is to break not three but five hours, for the distance. The "97-lb weakling" can develop a nicely formed body outline with a significant increase in strength. The uncoordinated large-size person can become a mistress of aerobic dance. But those people who do get somewhere previously unimagined almost invariably do so slowly, in a step-wise fashion, one step at a time. And they do so within their own body's limitations.

Thus the 400-lb man who would now require 67 minutes to walk a mile, can a year later be 100 lbs lighter, walking a mile in 30 minutes, and year after that, another 50 lbs lighter and walking a mile in 17 minutes. A formerly non-

---

THREE-MINUTE DRILL, 5 – 2

The Eight Elements of Taking Control

1. Understanding that motivation is not a thing, but a process that links a thought to a feeling with an action
2. Following the first four steps of the Wellness Motivational Process for Healthy Living from the beginning
3. Examining what one already does well; health-promoting behavioral changes already made
4. Recognizing that gradual change leads to permanent changes
5. Dealing with the fear both of failure and of success
6. The readiness to explore one's limits while recognizing one's limitations
7. Appreciating the process of psychological immediate gratification
8. Achieving balance, in the process of gradual change

athletic woman of normal weight can, after six months of training, be able to comfortably cover 20 miles on her bicycle in an hour and a half, and by the end of the following season ride her first century (100 miles) in nine hours, including a couple of stops for refreshment and rest. A 45-year-old with no background in running, cycling, or swimming can become a triathlete, finishing short-course races on a regular basis, happily and healthily towards the back-of-the-pack. The 97-lb weakling may become strong, but in his own terms, *e.g.,* being able to bench-press 120 lbs, not 275 lbs. And "well-formed" for this man will mean reducing his body-fat proportion to 18% from 25%, not the 4% of a professional body-builder. For our aerobic dancer, "mistress" may well mean that she is happy to regularly attend a one-hour class three times per week, doing the whole routine comfortably, at the instructor's pace, having gone from 40% overweight to 20% overweight. For her, it will not mean that she becomes a size six, with the ability to lead five classes a day, six days per week.

It is very important for you to be able to help patients recognize and accept their limitations. Speed, strength, muscular bulk, flexibility, gracefulness, are in part achieved through training and practice. But, as noted, they are in significant part achieved also as a result of genetic makeup. Exactly what proportion of each achievement is determined by one's genetic endowment and what proportion by one's own effort is of course not as yet known.

"Dealing with the fear of failure" means just what it says. Giving oneself permission to fail can be, for many, marvelously liberating and can actually help them significantly in navigating the pathway to success. There are many reasons for failure in becoming a regular exerciser, and it should be stressed that none of them have moral content. One is not a "Bad" person if one doesn't make it this time around. One can always try again, and if one never makes it, well, one just does not—and that should be the end of it, unless you and the patient are open to referral to another health professional who may be able, by taking a different tack of one kind or another, to ultimately achieve success. The necessity of dealing with the "fear of success" may come as a surprise, but this is a documented problem for certain persons, especially in the realm of weight-loss.

A THOUGHT ON "WILLPOWER"

In terms of personal health-related behavior change, the often misconstrued and misrepresented term, "willpower," **means:**

> The **conscious mental ability** to follow through on plans to make change and to maintain the change once it is made.

Defined in this way, willpower is essential if your patient is going to get on and stay on the Wellness Motivational Pathway. If anyone says that any health-promoting behavior change can be achieved without willpower, as defined here, he or she is blowing smoke. Yes, your patient does have to get organized to go through at least some version of the motivation-mobilizing process as it set forth in this chapter and the next. That takes focus, concentration, and commitment. That means mobilizing one's mental capacity to make a change in the carrying out of a physical act—nothing more and nothing less. That is precisely what the person changing her personal health-related behavior needs to do to make the desired change(s). (If you are planning to make major changes in the way you practice and/or in the way your practice setting is organized, you also need to mobilize your mental capacity in order to make those changes.) Yes, indeed, that does take willpower. It is that simple and that complicated.

References

1. Prochaska JO, Velicer WF. The transtheoretical model of behavior change. Am J Health Promot. 1997 Sept/Oct;12(1): 38–48.
2. Jonas S. Talking about training: stages of change, I. AMAA Q. 2000 Summer;17(2): 17.
3. Jonas S. Talking about training: stages of change, II. AMAA Q. 2000 Spring; 17(3):17.
4. Hilleboe HE, Barkhuus A, Thomas WC. Approaches to national health planning. In: Public health papers 46. Geneva (Switzerland): World Health Organization; 1972. p. 9–12.
5. Jonas S, Konner L. Just the weigh you are. Boston (MA): Chapters/Houghton Mifflin; 1997. 256 p.

CHAPTER 6

Mobilizing Motivation: Behavior Change Pyramid

Edward M. Phillips

OVERVIEW

As noted at the beginning of this book, there is more than one way to help patients to mobilize their motivation to make sustained lifestyle changes. In the last chapter we presented what might be called the "shorthand" version. In this chapter we present a more in-depth model. It is called the Behavior Change Pyramid. This model has been developed from evidenced-based principles of Motivational Interviewing, the Transtheoretical Model of Change (also discussed in Chapter 4), Behavioral Psychology, and the new field of coaching psychology. This model guides the clinician to perform more in-depth counseling of patients towards initiating and maintaining the habit of regular exercise, as well as for successfully making other health-promoting behavior changes.

The pyramidal structure of the model is intentional (Figure 6.1). At the foundation level, the patient is asked to create a *Vision* of a life that includes regular exercise. To make this a sustained lifestyle change, the patient needs to grapple with the fundamental issues of taking *responsibility* for the proposed change, completing an inventory of personal *strengths,* coming to grips with the higher purpose or personal *values* to be met by adopting a more active lifestyle, and developing planning *strategies* to overcome predictable *obstacles.* Lastly, the patient is responsible for gathering information and education about the *benefits* and indeed the *risks* of becoming more active.

At the second level of the process, the patient is still dynamically thinking and planning and has not yet taken a definitive action, such as joining a gym. At this *Preparation* stage the *Vision* is transformed into a realistic plan. The patient garners the necessary *support* to allow the time and achieve access to exercise along with people on her support team, assesses her *confidence* level in adopting and maintaining a new physical activity program, makes a verbal or written *commitment* to cement her resolve, and creates a series of achievable *goals and plans* toward the eventual objective.

Interestingly, it is not until the third level of the pyramid that it is recommended to the patient to take any definitive *Action.* Planning and thinking lay the foundation for successfully making behavior change. All too often patients

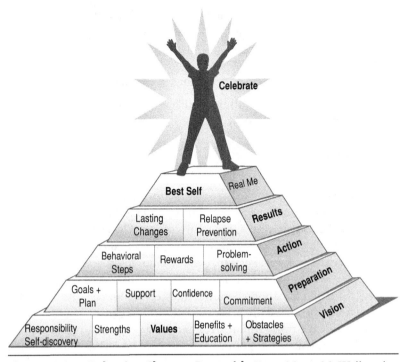

Figure 6.1 • Behavior Change Pyramid. From Moore M. Wellcoaches manual. Philadelphia: Lippincott Williams & Wilkins. 2009, p. 43.

resolve to quickly change from a sedentary or nearly inactive lifestyle to one that includes daily vigorous exercise. This sudden change from sedentary to vigorous activity is a recipe for post-exercise pain and injury that often leads to resentment, frustration, and quitting. Also, without the necessary planning the patient has no means of support or an alternative pathway to follow should he become injured or run into other obstacles. Once the patient addresses the first two levels of *Vision* and *Preparation,* he can take the first *behavioral steps* of, say, joining a gym, starting another type of exercise program or joining a class or team. At the same time, it is reasonable to start to experiment with exercise, such as walking, alongside the thinking and planning work.

In the *Action* phase, *rewards* ideally are contemplated and created, but delayed until there is feedback on the first actions. At this *Action* level the patient now works to learn brainstorming and *problem-solving* strategies for dealing with unanticipated obstacles such as an injury or inclement weather.

At the fourth level, *Results,* the patient prepares a back up plan for dealing with possible *relapses.* At this level the patient learns to incorporate the behavior change as a *lasting change* or habit in her regular routine. At the fifth and final level, the patient has the opportunity to incorporate the new exercise routine into her evolving concept of *The Best Self.* The fulfilled original value established in the base level is supported by the success.

Patient Vignette

Let's bring this model to life by considering this patient:

- 44 year old mother of two, full time office manager
- Mild hypertension
- BMI = 28
- No medications
- Sedentary

Your patient decides to take *responsibility* for a plan to no longer be sedentary. She identifies as a *strength* her ability to plan ahead. This is the same strength that she uses as a manager in her office. The *value* of being a good role model for her young children is elicited. As a clinician, you explain the *benefits* of increased physical activity in bringing down your patient's blood pressure. Her *obstacle* of not liking to be uncomfortable during exercise is addressed through education about the marked health benefits of moderate physical activity through daily brisk walks (without getting out of breath).

Setting aside the thirty minutes for her daily walk requires the *support* of her coworkers and husband. Your patient expresses very low *confidence* in her ability to immediately reach her ultimate goal of doing 30 minutes of physical activity each day, but has a high level of confidence (8 out of 10) that she can achieve an initial goal of 10 minutes of daily physical activity. Your patient's *commitment* to walk with a coworker 10 minutes every day at lunch is cemented by a written agreement signed and included in her medical record. The *goals and plan* are detailed in your written exercise prescription.

With all of this critical planning and thinking in place, the *active* next step of commencing her daily lunchtime walks flows seamlessly. As part of the original plan, she *rewards* herself with a new pair of sneakers after adhering to her daily walks for a full month. *Problem-solving* skills are called into play when her walking buddy is away from work for several days. During this time she tries listening to music during her walks. After three months of daily walks, your patient begins to incorporate the habit of daily walks as a *lasting change.* However, when her coworker is transferred to another office, your patient *relapses* toward inactivity. She reviews her relapse plan and her original *values and goals* for becoming active. She is also more aware that she feels sluggish and irritable when she skips her walking. She becomes a role model for her children and introduces a new coworker to the daily lunchtime walks. In this ideal progression, your patient moves along in an orderly fashion toward a more physically active lifestyle. The same Behavior Change Pyramid can be applied to dealing with other lifestyle behavior changes addressing, for example, nutrition, weight management, stress management, or tobacco use.

It should be noted that however simply we present this model, your patient's experience is not likely to be so straightforward. For most people, behavior change does not follow a linear pathway in which one proceeds from the bottom directly to the top of the pyramid. Your patients can cycle up and down the five levels sometimes for years before incorporating a lasting change into what finally becomes their new self-concept. On the other hand, some simple health-promoting behaviors such as drinking two extra glasses of water per day may be quickly incorporated.

The Behavior Change Pyramid can also be used to determine the missing or weak building block that undid a prior attempt to become active. Your patient will commonly report prior periods of physical activity that ended with the onset of poor weather (not planning for *obstacles*), progressing too quickly in a running program and becoming injured (not adhering to a *plan* for small steps), or actually achieving the original *value* such as becoming fit for a special event and then having no reason to continue exercising after that achievement.

Now that we have covered the general principles of the Behavior Change Pyramid, let's address in more detail the particular issues that can arise at each stage of the process and how the clinician can help patients to initiate and maintain an active lifestyle.

VISION LEVEL

Self-Responsibility

This concept is deceptively simple to both the clinician and the patient. In the predominant model of medical care, the clinician is the expert. In a life-threatening emergency, for example, the clinician is appropriately entrusted to, hopefully, save the patient's life. Lifestyle change, however, occurs in the context of myriad small decisions made by the patient throughout the day. The clinician is not there, for example, to remind the patient to use the stairs or to go to the gym after work. This gateway of *self-responsibility* into the Behavior Change Model is strategically placed because it provides the opportunity to triage the patient's level of readiness for making the proposed change.

At the outset, the *self-responsibility* box of the pyramid screens for those patients who are *ready, willing, and able* to commit to making a series of small changes in their daily physical activity level. To be successful your patient must, with your guidance, take personal responsibility for determining *what* change she will make, *when* she will do this, and *why* she will alter her current habits. To be successful, the patient needs to internalize the responsibility for change, rather than look externally for a quick fix, such as the latest exercise gadget advertised on television that guarantees a weight loss of 20 pounds in 4 weeks.

If your patient is not yet ready to take responsibility for making a certain behavior change in one way, he may be willing to take responsibility for making such a change in a different way. For example, the patient may not yet be ready to take responsibility for setting aside the time for leisure-time scheduled exercise, but may be able to commit to the lifestyle approach of slowly increasing the amount of physical activity he does during the course of the day. However, if the patient is not ready to accept responsibility for making any change at the current time, as the clinician you can still provide support and helpful information, such as the benefits of physical activity for his particular circumstance, which may help him to make the desired change somewhere down the road.

This initial block on the Behavior Change Pyramid also presents the clinician with the opportunity to share the responsibility with the patient. You will appropriately advise and coach your patient toward a lifetime of regular exercise; however, your patient will rightfully need to assume the expert role in determining what strategies will most likely support this transition, for him- or herself. As we discussed in Chapter 2, not all clinicians will be comfortable with making this transition.

Providing your patient with a written exercise prescription utilizes your authority as an expert to recommend the best course of action to your patients. It also presents them with a health-promoting behavior change recommendation in a form that they are familiar with as coming from a clinician: the Prescription. The art and science of behavior change counseling as it is presently understood tells us that it is best done when a) the patient becomes an active partner in the decision-making process and b) when that process is codified with the written prescription. For lifestyle behavior-change recommendations, its use can be most valuable for any clinician, even those clinicians not accustomed or licensed to write prescriptions for medications. Writing an exercise prescription for the otherwise healthy patient can be most helpful, in both codifying the recommendation(s) and giving them weight. (In Chapter 3, Risk Assessment and Exercise Screening, we address the situation of those patients who need further evaluation by a physician or exercise testing before initiating an exercise program.)

Strengths

In order to motivate your patients to adopt and adhere to an exercise program, it is useful to help them understand the strengths that have helped them achieve other goals. For example, a patient who has completed advanced schooling may be reminded of the discipline that it took to achieve his degree. The clinician's role is augmented by focusing on the patient's strengths rather than attempting to correct the patient's weaknesses. This approach enables the patient to rise above and outgrow his problems. You may simply ask your patient, "What are your strengths and how can you use them to support your exercise program?" A self-generated list of strengths will be vital for the patient to overcome obstacles and problems along the path of regular exercise.

Values

The clinician or coach working with a patient needs to help her explore her core values to determine the higher purpose of becoming more active. As a trusted clinician you may be instrumental in guiding patients to discovering their enduring core values that will mobilize their motivation. For example, a 41-year-old married nurse and daughter of a parent with dementia reports that in fulfilling her primary value and role as a caregiver, she puts the needs of others before her own. As such she never gets around to exercising because her parents and patients need her attention. The clinician can help her understand that caring for herself by increasing daily physical activity will make her healthier, more energetic, less irritable and, consequently, a better and more consistent caregiver for others. You are giving the patient permission to value self-care highly and recognize that it is the foundation for being their best at home and at work.

Helping patients explore and prioritize their underlying purpose in adhering to an exercise program, the clinician may need to probe beyond the first answer by asking, "What's so great about that?" This may lead to a more substantial value and move beyond more superficial values such as looking good. While becoming fit for an appearance at a specific event, such as a wedding, may provide great motivation until the event has passed, a more enduring value of maintaining balance in life and improving self-esteem may help the patient maintain the exercise program over the long-term. This also changes the focus from immediate results of a new exercise program to starting the process of fulfilling the values and reaching toward the *Best Self.* The value that the patient holds in adhering to an exercise program will be revisited when problems arise or when the patient has lapsed from the program. At the same time, having an event-specific goal as the first one can help the patient to get started, with the realization that their mental resources will need to be re-mobilized if they are going to be able to stay with it.

List of Values for Regular Exercise:

- Looking good or youthful
- Being a role model
- Having peace of mind
- Reducing stress
- Building self-esteem
- Being in control
- Feeling more healthy
- Having more energy
- Losing weight
- Maintaining independence (older adults)

Benefits and Education

As noted in the Introduction, there is no shortage of public health pronouncements, articles in popular magazines, television interviews, and medical literature extolling the dramatic benefits of physical activity. The simple question is, "If exercise is so great, why don't more people do it?" One answer is that the patient has not yet tilted the *decisional balance* of his motivations and rewards of remaining inactive versus the motivation and rewards of adopting regular exercise. In this instance, the clinician has the opportunity to personalize the benefits of exercise to the unique medical and family history and circumstances of the patient. Indeed, without the explicit personalized advice and prescription of a trusted healthcare professional, the simple knowledge that exercise is beneficial in general may continue to be ignored by the patient. The patient's concerns and motivations will tilt the *decisional balance* toward either inactivity or exercise. Taking this a step further, the failure to prescribe exercise may be perceived as a tacit endorsement of the patient's inactivity, thereby tilting the balance away from exercise.

This box in the foundation of the pyramid is perhaps the most important site for clinicians to intervene. Personalizing the benefits of exercise to the patients will help them identify, explore, prioritize, and emotionally connect to the potential benefits from becoming and maintaining regular physical activity.

Obstacles and Strategies

Before initiating or increasing physical activity, the patient must enumerate the known major obstacles to his plan as part of the critical thinking and planning process. For example, if the patient commits to walking 10–15 minutes after dinner each night in his neighborhood, it is reasonable to foresee the obstacle of bad weather occurring and to plan specific strategies for dealing with it. This may include a switch to walking at an indoor mall, or on a treadmill at home, or in a gym. This process calls for articulating realistic strategies to deal with known obstacles. It is critical that the patient has confidence in the strategy. In some cases, the excitement of initiating a new exercise program will make the obstacles seem to fade away. Even so, it is prudent to plan ahead for obstacles when the initial enthusiasm subsides. Overcoming the obstacle of lack of time to exercise may be reduced by the strategy of using a gym at work, at home, or within a 10-minute drive. Moreover, incorporating lifestyle exercise into a daily routine will be less time-intrusive than scheduled leisure-time exercise. These strategies will support your patient when other priorities arise.

The following list of obstacles to engaging in a regular exercise program may start with whatever derailed the patient in her prior attempts to begin and maintain a regular exercise program.

Common Obstacles to Regular Exercise:

Lack of time	Lack of interest
Other priorities	Prefer relaxing
Lack of confidence	Perceived benefits of remaining
Lack of money to join a gym, buy	inactive
equipment or appropriate clothing	Fear of injury
Don't want to be sweaty or uncomfortable	Change in routine
Boredom	Lack of support from family or job
Pain or injury	Don't know what exercise to do
"I'm too old."	Adverse weather

SUMMARY OF THE VISION LEVEL

At this foundation level, the patient takes responsibility for becoming more physically active and explores her underlying values for becoming a regular exerciser. The decision to make a change is influenced by the clinician who personalizes the benefits of exercise to the patient. That is, the clinician helps the patient understand the *pros* for change versus the obstacles or *cons* for change. Developing strategies to overcome the obstacles helps to tip the balance toward more physical activity and to lay the foundation for lasting change.

PREPARATION LEVEL

Commitment

Your patient's dedication to a new exercise program is formalized when he offers his verbal and/or written commitment to follow through on the exercise prescription. The detailed nature of the exercise prescription allows him to specifically state exactly what he plans to do. For example, an 84-year-old retired chemist has investigated the benefits of strength training and a modest walking program to maintain his independence in his own home. He is motivated, but never seems to get around to starting the exercise program. He makes an oral commitment in your office to initiate his exercise program, agrees to sign his written exercise vision and plan filed in his medical record, and sends weekly progress reports to your office. This formalized commitment on his part supports his new exercise regimen and makes him accountable. His high level of integrity and habit of honoring his commitments helps mobilize him into action.

Support

The 44-year-old woman introduced in the first vignette needs to obtain the support of her coworkers for the daily 30 minutes of walking that she plans. On the weekend, her husband watches the children while she goes for her walks. He also encourages her to continue this new habit when she starts to get bored. Indeed, the husband begins to join her on the weekend walks while a neighbor watches the children. Your provision of an exercise prescription to your patient is another critical form of support. The prescription helps her overcome her fear of injury from the activity by detailing the slow, steady, safe increase of activity. Her walking buddy provides social support, companionship, and shared commitment to their joint goal. When the walking buddy is transferred to another office and the patient lapses into inactivity, it is her children who question why she stopped walking and they push her to resume.

Just as the Exercise Prescription is very specific, it is helpful for your patients to be as explicit as possible about who is on their support team and what type of support they need to make their regular exercise a reality.

Support Structures:

Spouse
Significant Other
Family
Friends
Supervisor/coworkers
Work site program
Online community
Class in School
Religious Group
Social Group
Personal Trainer
Wellness Coach
Physician
Health Care Practitioner
Financial Support:
    Work site incentive programs
Health insurance incentive programs

Access to an environment conducive
    to exercise:
Home
Gym
Fitness club
Park space/safe neighborhood
Community center

Types of Support:
Financial support
Time away from work or home
    responsibilities
Encouragement
Positive feedback
Companionship
Inspiration/motivation from others

Confidence

As your patients set out on the road to becoming regular exercisers, it is vital that they have sufficient *self-efficacy* or "confidence to sustain the behavior in the face of their obstacles." Confidence plays a critical role in making any sort of behavior change. For your patient to be successful in adopting a new behavior such as regular exercise, he will need a moderate to high level of confidence in his ability to accomplish the goal. To determine your patient's level of confidence in the proposed change, *e.g.,* lifting weights for 15 minutes twice per week, you can simply ask the patient to rate his confidence on a scale of 1–10.

If he rates his confidence level less than 7 out of 10, then he needs to either reduce the magnitude of the proposed change or to raise his confidence levels.

For example, your patient may report a confidence level of 4 out of 10 when asked if he can reliably begin a program of 30 minutes of brisk walking daily, but a confidence level of 9 out of 10 if the initial prescription is for only 10 minutes of daily walking. One of the tenets of behavior change is using small steps and setting achievable goals. While 10 minutes of daily walking is below the recommended physical activity guidelines, accomplishing this initial goal improves the patient's health and, importantly, raises his confidence to achieve other behavior changes.

As we discussed in the section on *Self-Responsibility,* your role as the expert may undermine the patient's sense of self-efficacy. When the patient takes responsibility for her health behaviors and begins to achieve small goals, she gains the confidence to become an authority over her own health. You will play an instrumental role in marking the progress of your patient and helping to improve her confidence by listing the goals achieved to that point.

Goals and Plan

The exercise prescription negotiated with the patient provides a Specific, Measurable, Achievable, Realistic, and Time-Bound (SMART) goal for the patient to pursue. This is better than a vague recommendation to "get more exercise." In filling the prescription, the patient will track his performance and participation in a log, journal, Web site, or automatically through attendance at an exercise class. These goals and plan will be updated periodically when the patient revisits or reports his progress. It is natural, as initial physical fitness and performance goals are achieved, to expand the goal so that the brisk walk becomes a run or other more vigorous activity.

Patients will be more successful if they plan ahead for their scheduled leisure-time exercise or are continually mindful of opportunities to increase their lifestyle exercise like taking the stairs instead of the elevator or walking instead of driving to the store.

SUMMARY OF PREPARATION LEVEL

At this second level of the pyramid, planning for regular exercise continues. The patient's confidence level is assessed and specific, achievable goals are set that will enable success. Your patients seek out the support structure to enable them to become more active. A written or oral commitment cements their resolve.

ACTION LEVEL

Behavioral Steps

As your patients begin to fill the exercise prescription, they are finally progressing from the thinking and planning steps to taking action. Because of prior preparation, the patient will be taking action that is safe and sustainable. Instead of responding to a New Year's resolution to get into shape and suddenly go from inactivity to daily gym classes, the patient is starting with small, manageable, but challenging steps. Their risk of injury is diminished and their self-efficacy is improved by initial successes.

Patients' progress will vary from week to week, but reviewing their activity logs or pedometer readings will help track the longer trend as the new habit of regular exercise develops.

To solidify the new habit of regular exercise, the patient will need to consistently commit to an initial three months of physical activity and then maintain the activity for an additional three months. At this point, the exercise becomes part of her regular routine and missing the activity is the exception rather than the norm.

Problem Solving

When we first addressed *obstacles and strategies* on the vision level as part of the foundation for change, patients were led through tactics for dealing with known or expected major impediments. Yet patients will inevitably encounter unplanned challenges and setbacks to starting and maintaining regular exercise. The process of problem solving calls for brainstorming to modify the original exercise prescription, adjusting expectations, and looking for opportunities to learn and grow despite the hindrance. Through the problem solving process, patients understand that impediments invariably arise and that being flexible enables them to experiment with new strategies that may present other opportunities.

For example, the dedicated runner presenting to your office with a leg injury may need to postpone his planned road race and modify his exercise regimen to temporarily avoid running. Instead, he follows an alternative exercise prescription that includes swimming, core strengthening, upper extremity strengthening, and a more aggressive stretching program. He exercises on a stationery bicycle while his leg heals. The newly added exercises become incorporated into a rotation of activities when the patient resumes his running and he proceeds to his first triathlon.

The experience of successfully adapting to one problem improves your patient's confidence and expectation that he will clear the next hurdle that comes along.

Rewards

Once the *Action* step has begun and your patient is becoming physically active, it is important for your patient to experience early rewards to reinforce motivation and confidence. Some of the rewards come directly as a result of the exercise: feeling better, looking better, becoming stronger and more energetic, having improved self-esteem, and being in control. While it is a good idea to observe, enjoy, and celebrate the rewards of the new exercise program, it is important to have appropriate rewards. One of the challenges of initiating an exercise program is that the physiologic changes of exercise take several weeks or months to be noticed. Interestingly, the effects of resistance training resulting in increased weightlifting capacity will be evidenced within several weeks of commencing the program, while cardiovascular exercise will take longer to achieve noticeable changes. Therefore, patients may respond to the reward of recognition of their accomplishments by their clinician. Further, the clinician is in an advantageous position to document and give feedback on the tangible results of the increased activity on their improved health status: decreased blood lipids, decreased body fat measurements, improved functional capacity, etc.

SUMMARY OF ACTION LEVEL

After all the thinking and planning levels, taking action follows. As interim small goals are achieved, rewards are taken. Flexibility to deal with problems along the road is employed.

RESULTS LEVEL

Lasting Change

As noted previously the difficult part of regular exercise is the *regular,* not the exercise. By this point your patient has adopted a new habit and describes a high level of confidence in continuing for the foreseeable future. To sustain this change the initial extrinsic motivation (including your exercise prescription) now has to become a more sustainable intrinsic motivation. Patients are more in touch with how pleasurable it is to be physically active on a regular basis. This is the point where patients may begin to express that *not* exercising feels bad to them.

It takes 3–6 months to establish a new exercise behavior or habit, and once the habit has been sustained for an additional six months, we can declare success, and encourage patients to be continually vigilant about staying on track. It is helpful to explore and savor all of the ramifications and benefits of this new habit.

Relapse Prevention

In order to sustain a new behavior, it is important to consider current challenges and to revisit, as appropriate, all of the building blocks of the Behavior Change Pyramid to ensure that the structure supporting lasting change continues to be robust. Encouraging patients to become role models and to help others can be an important new self-image and motivator.

Despite the best intentions of your patients to continue exercising regularly, they may stop due to injury, competing time commitments, boredom, etc. Relapse is so common that it is helpful to expect this to occur and to plan for it. Simply understanding how common it is to lapse from an exercise program will help your patient to get back on track when this occurs. The patient will do well to revisit the original values enumerated in the foundation to recall the core motivators for becoming physically active. Restarting the exercise program and remembering that any regular exercise is healthier than no extra physical activity at all will help direct the patient. Other building blocks along the way may be revisited, *e.g.,* reconnecting with the support structure or reviewing the strategies to overcome obstacles.

SUMMARY OF RESULTS LEVEL

The new habit of exercising is sustained by intrinsic motivation. Planning for relapse helps patients from sliding back into inactivity.

BEST SELF

The process of behavior change helps your patient evolve to a healthier state and to get closer to his ideal self. It is a journey of personal growth. You have helped your patient to uncover her athletic or active self or to at least adopt a regular pattern of walking or some other physical activity that she enjoys. When your patients experience being their best selves, they are energized, more positive, and confident. Acknowledge their transformations enthusiastically and find creative ways to help them celebrate their successes.

SUMMARY

While the journey of behavior change is challenging and requires a lot of thinking, planning, and acting, the opportunities to encourage and inspire your patients to be the best that they can be and to witness their growth will soon become some of your most rewarding work.

Suggested Reading

Bandura A. Self-efficacy: the exercise of control. New York: W. H. Freeman & Company; 1997. 604 p.

Bandura A. Self-efficacy: toward unifying theory of behavioral change. Psychol Rev. 1997 Mar;84(2):191–215.

Bandura A. Social foundations of thought and action: a social cognitive theory. Englewood Cliffs, NJ: Prentice Hall; 1986. 544 p.

Botelho R. Motivate healthy habits: stepping stones to lasting change. Rochester, NY: MHH Publications; 2004. 160 p.

Botelho R. Motivational practice: promoting healthy habits and self-care for chronic disease Rochester, NY: MHH Publications; 2004. 336 p.

Deutschman A. Change or die: the three keys to change at work and in life. New York: HarperCollins Publishers; 2007. 256 p.

Janis IL, Mann L. Decision making: a psychological analysis of conflict, choice, and commitment. New York: The Free Press; 1977. 488 p.

Miller WR, Rollnick S. Motivational interviewing: preparing people for change. New York: Guilford Press; 2002. 428 p.

Moore M. Wellcoaches manual. Philadelphia: Lippincott Williams & Wilkins. 2009.

Prochaska JO, Norcross J, DiClemente C. Changing for good: A revolutionary six-stage program for overcoming bad habits and moving your life positively forward. New York: William Morrow Publishing; 1994. 304 p.

Willis J, Campbell LF. Exercise psychology. Champaign, IL: Human Kinetics; 1992. 344 p.

CHAPTER 7

Getting Started as a Regular Exerciser

Edward M. Phillips, Jennifer Capell, and Steven Jonas

INTRODUCTION

By this stage of the book, you will have most likely come to the understanding that the hardest part of becoming and staying a regular exerciser is the mental work that has to be done at all the stages of the process: getting ready to begin, becoming active, and then staying with it. In the previous three chapters, we have dealt with the central mental task: mobilizing motivation and keeping it activated. In this chapter we will deal with additional mental aspects of getting started, whether your patient is going to try the lifestyle exercise approach or the leisure-time scheduled exercise approach, whether it be a sport such as running or an athletic activity such as aerobic dance.

Remember, if all that people needed were advice on what sports to do, and when to do them, we would have a nation of regular exercisers, and this book would be unnecessary. However, observation and research tell us that the majority of successful regular exercisers have spent a significant amount of time mentally preparing and engaging in their activity: thinking about what they are going to do and why they are going to do it. They use approaches on the order of either the Wellness Motivational Pathway (Chapter 5) or the Behavior Change Pyramid (Chapter 6). Further, we have suggested that you strongly advise your patient to take some time to think about what she is going to do and why she wants to do it, to write down her thoughts, and to then carefully consider what she has written even before taking that first step.

The process of assisting your patient in moving from a sedentary lifestyle to an active one can be broken down into three stages: the Foundation Phase, the Becoming Active Phase, and the Staying Active Phase. As you have discovered in the previous chapters of this book, a fair amount of the "work" involved with getting active happens before your patient begins his first "workout." These pre-activity components, including progressing through the Stages of Change by the patient, screening and professional assessment to determine readiness for regular exercise and exercise risk for the patient, and Mobilizing Motivation make up Phase I, the Foundation Phase. These topics have been covered in Chapters 3–6.

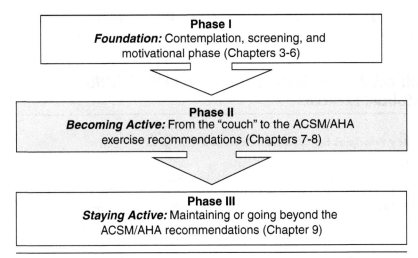

Figure 7.1 • The Phases of Lifestyle Change: From Sedentary to Active

Once your patient has been adequately prepared to begin an exercise program, she enters Phase II, the Becoming Active Phase. In this phase, your patient will progress from a sedentary state up to the ACSM/AHA recommended minimal exercise levels (1). This phase is the focus of the present chapter and the next, and part of Chapter 10. Finally, once your patient has reached the nationally recommended minimum and has maintained it for some period of time (and has been sufficiently congratulated by you for doing so!), she will progress to Phase III, the Staying Active Phase, the topic of Chapter 9 and part of Chapter 10. In this phase, she will have a choice to maintain her current level at or above the ACSM/AHA minimum recommendations, or to safely progress to an even more active lifestyle. Figure 7.1 illustrates the three phases of lifestyle change from sedentary to active.

As we move into the actual prescription of exercise, we will present two options: the general principles of exercise prescription, which should enable you to prescribe a personalized program for your patients, and a specific program. The generalized principles are covered in Chapters 8 and 9, while the specific program is the topic of Chapter 10.

Although Figure 7.1 shows a linear progression through the three phases, patients can and will move between the phases over time. For example, motivation will periodically wane in all individuals, requiring the patient, with our without your assistance, to remobilize his motivation. Similarly, a patient who has reached Phase III could regress back to the ACSM/AHA minimum recommended levels, or even back to the sedentary level. In such situations, remind your patient that: a) every regular exerciser experiences such variations, at one level or another; b) he has not "failed," or is a not a "bad" person for doing so;

and c) when he is ready to do so, you will be there to encourage him to return to whatever the appropriate phase, and start progressing again.

THE KEY PRINCIPLES FOR SUCCESSFULLY PRESCRIBING REGULAR EXERCISE

Key Principles for Successful Exercise Prescription

1. Set "SMART" goals
2. Focus first on the "regular" in "regular exercise"
3. Gradual change lead to permanent changes
4. More is better than less, but something is better than nothing

Set "SMART" Goals

As we have discussed earlier, it is critical that your patient has a well-defined goal(s) that she is working toward. As with any goal, your patient's active lifestyle goals should follow the "SMART" (*Specific, Measurable, Attainable, Realistic,* and *Time-Bound*) formula. These points will be elaborated upon as we proceed. We encourage you to write your patient's goal(s) on her Exercise Prescription to ensure that, together, you have determined the goal(s). This then becomes a handy reminder for your patient as she progresses toward the goal(s). Some patients do set multiple goals for themselves, which can be helpful in both mobilizing and maintaining motivation. As we have noted more than once, when setting a goal, your patient should consider questions such as what the primary reason(s) is for becoming more active: Why is this important? What do I expect to get out of the activity? Am I prepared to make the adjustments in lifestyle in order to reach the goal? (See Figure 7.2.)

Focus First on the "Regular" in "Regular Exercise"

Patients will have the greatest chance of success if they focus first on the "regular" component, rather than on the "exercise" component of "regular exercise." Assuming that the mental preparation and planning have been done appropriately, we recommend that your patient begin by focusing first on developing the habit of regular exercise by building the time for exercise, whether in the lifestyle or the leisure-time scheduled approach, into their life on a regular basis. Before your patient can succeed at committing to any given activity, he needs to convince himself that he can do it on a regular basis. The ACSM and AHA recommend that adults be moderately physically active for 30 minutes at least five days a week, or for 20 minutes at least three days each week if participating in vigorous exercise. Moderate-intensity exercise is

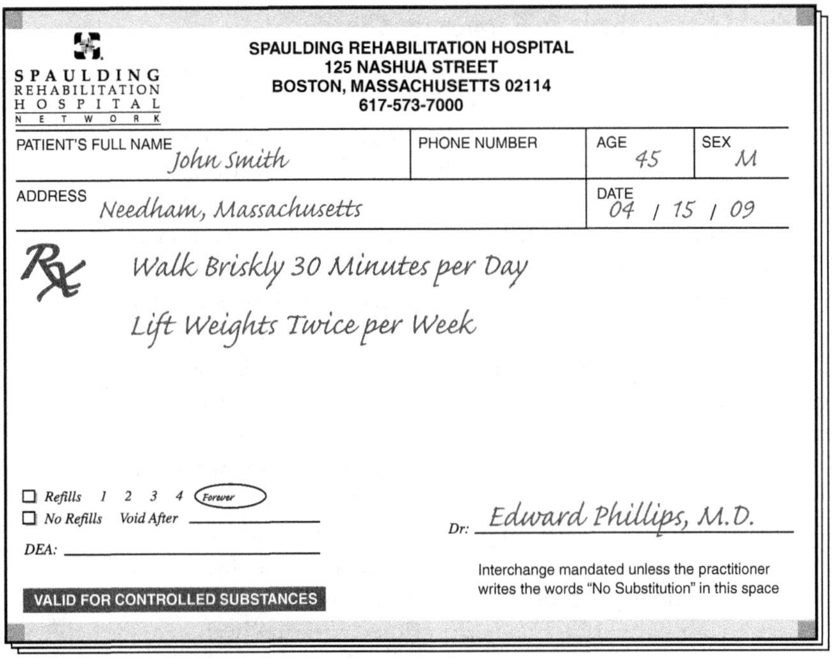

	SPAULDING REHABILITATION HOSPITAL			
	125 NASHUA STREET			
S P A U L D I N G	BOSTON, MASSACHUSETTS 02114			
R E H A B I L I T A T I O N	617-573-7000			
H O S P I T A L				
N E T W O R K				

| PATIENT'S FULL NAME | PHONE NUMBER | AGE | SEX |
| *John Smith* | | *45* | *M* |

| ADDRESS | DATE |
| *Needham, Massachusetts* | *04 / 15 / 09* |

$\mathrm{R}_{\!X}$ *Walk Briskly 30 Minutes per Day*

Lift Weights Twice per Week

☐ *Refills   1   2   3   4   Forever*
☐ *No Refills   Void After* _____

DEA: _____

Dr: *Edward Phillips, M.D.*

VALID FOR CONTROLLED SUBSTANCES

Interchange mandated unless the practitioner
writes the words "No Substitution" in this space

Figure 7.2 • A very basic exercise goal handwritten on prescription pad: "Walk 30 minutes at least five days per week."

defined as working hard enough to noticeably increase heart rate and breathing, yet still being able to carry on a conversation, and vigorous exercise is activity that substantially increases heart rate and breathing. Vigorous-intensity exercise is formally defined as >60% $\dot{V}O_2$ R. See Chapter 8 for a more extensive discussion of exercise intensity (2). In addition, it is important to discuss the regularity, or distribution, of activity throughout the week. It is preferable for your patients to try to distribute their activity sessions throughout the week, rather than fitting all activity into the weekend, for example. An even distribution, especially as the activity level increases, is less likely to cause overuse injury, can help increase metabolism for a greater period of time over the course of the week, and provides a greater benefit for both the heart and skeletal muscles. In the non-conditioned person, intermittent episodes of a significantly increased heart rate can increase the risk of sudden death from heart attack. These heart rate increases may result from activities such as climbing several flights of stairs quickly while carrying a heavy briefcase. With respect to the musculoskeletal system, muscles worked out on a regular basis, on alternate days at least, go through a cycle of build-up, breakdown, and further build-up. This process leads to increased endurance and strength.

Gradual Change Leads to Permanent Changes

Being sedentary or being active is a habit. Habits are hard to break. Changing a sedentary habit into an active habit will take time and is best tackled in small increments. In Chapter 8 you will learn how to actually prescribe exercise for your patients as you might prescribe any other health-related intervention, and to help them maintain or progress their exercise program over time.

In this process, you will help your patient to determine a starting point that does not seem overwhelming or difficult to her, and from there, to progress by small amounts each week. This approach decreases the chance of overuse injury and increases the chances of success in changing her sedentary habit into an active habit. For most people, "too much, too soon," whether in the lifestyle or leisure-time scheduled approach, will lead to muscle pain and possible injury, as well as to greater likelihood of early quitting. Furthermore, a series of small, "doable," changes will soon result in big changes. A few weeks or months into the program, your patient will likely look back at the extent of her progress, and be surprised but motivated and proud of her accomplishments.

The encouraging news is that just as a sedentary habit is hard to break but can be done if done gradually, an active habit is also hard to break—meaning that once your patient has made the effort to gradually change his habit and to incorporate regular activity into his lifestyle, it will be significantly easier to maintain this new way of life. In fact, he will most likely even enjoy the benefits of the exercise!

More Is Better than Less, but Something Is Better than Nothing

Throughout this book, we recommend that your patients strive to reach and maintain an exercise level of at least 150 minutes of moderate-intensity physical activity, or 60 minutes of vigorous-intensity exercise each week—the recommendations established by the ACSM and AHA. The benefits of physical activity increase with the amount of activity performed, because of the dose-response relationship between exercise and the health benefits accrued from the exercise. Therefore, as your patients begin and progress through their exercise program, they should be encouraged to keep increasing at a safe rate of progression at least until they reach the national minimal recommended levels.

The relative risk of all-cause mortality declines sharply from a sedentary patient who is active for only 30 minutes per week (point A, Figure 7.3), but flattens out after achieving approximately 150 minutes (2.5 hours) of moderate to vigorous leisure-time activity per week (point C, Figure 7.3). Note that additional activity beyond the 2.5 hours confers greater benefits. These findings help form the basis of the minimum recommendation of 150 minutes per week of moderate-intensity physical activity, with the recommendation that greater activity confers greater benefits (points D and E, Figure 7.3). The recommended activity levels can be translated into caloric expenditures on a weekly basis. The average person walking 3 miles per hour burns approximately 100 kcal

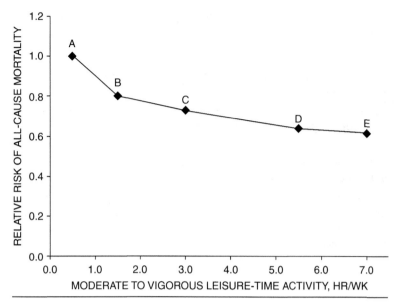

Figure 7.3 • "Median" Shape of the Dose-Response Curve
Source: http://www.health.gov/paguidelines/Report/G1_allcause.aspx#q3

per mile or 300 kcal per hour. At the recommended 150 minutes (or 2.5 hours per week), your patient will expend approximately 750 kcal in physical activity per week. The general goal of 1,000 to 2,000 kcal of energy expenditure per week assists with maintaining weight loss and improving longevity (3, 4). To achieve the energy expenditure in these ranges, your patient will need to exercise at higher intensity or for longer than the minimum recommendations. These minimum levels, however, may seem unreachable to some patients. We encourage you to gently "push" your patients to become more active—in whatever capacity they are able. This may mean beginning with tiny steps toward a more active lifestyle. These steps should be greatly encouraged and positively reinforced, even if the patient is not yet ready to commit to striving to reach the ACSM/AHA recommendations. In short, a positive step would be to engage your patient in discussing and contemplating becoming more active. As illustrated in Figure 7.3, even at levels below the minimum recommendations there are general health benefits of additional activity. On the other end of the curve, the general health benefits of exercise no longer increase after approximately 3,500 to 4,000 kcal (7 to 10 hours) of exercise per week. Using the metaphor of exercise as medicine, this level represents the *ceiling effect* for general health benefits. Those patients who wish to train at more intense levels or for longer periods of time per week will, however, continue to accrue higher levels of fitness. An *overdose* of exercise or overtraining may become an issue for the rare patient.

In Chapter 9 we address the safe progression of exercise, as well as the topic of overtraining.

HELPING YOUR PATIENTS INCORPORATE EXERCISE INTO THEIR LIFESTYLE

Committing to Making the Time to Exercise

Ways to Minimize the Amount of "Extra" Time that Physical Activity Takes:
- Add exercise into current activities (*e.g.,* park in the open spots at the far end of the parking lot and walk, or take the stairs instead of waiting for the elevator)
- Combine activity and socializing—meet for a walk rather than for coffee
- Identify "wasted time" during the day, and fill it with physical activity

It is unavoidable that becoming a regular exerciser will take time out of the rest of your patient's schedule for the rest of her life. To become a regular exerciser, your patient must recognize and accept this. This does not, however, need to be negatively construed. First, by incorporating exercise into daily activities, such as finding a parking spot at the far end of the parking lot and walking a little farther, the time commitment does not have to be as great as your patient may initially think. Other ways of minimizing the amount of extra time that exercise takes up include planning ahead and using currently "wasted time," or combining socializing and exercising. In the latter option, for example, your patient could meet a friend for a walk rather than for coffee, or plan to get the coffee *after* the walk. It is important, however, to make sure that your patient is scheduling in extra time for exercise, or is thinking of concrete ways in which she can incorporate regular moderate physical activity into her daily activities.

Second, considering the numerous health benefits (see Chapter 1) of developing an active lifestyle, having your patient commit to 150 minutes—or less if she is willing and able to exercise at a *vigorous* intensity—is a small price to pay for realizing such great benefits. Finally, although the time commitment may seem great at the start of his exercise program, it is likely that he will soon adjust and even start looking forward to exercising and the way it makes him feel. Individuals who move to a home further away from their work may initially find the added commuting time annoying, but will likely soon become accustomed to the new use of time. Adding exercise time into a daily routine is similar—your patient will soon become accustomed to the change. With exercise however, your patient will also gain all the added benefits of improved mental and physical health. Central to maintaining the commitment to exercise is appropriate motivation and goal-setting. To assist your patient with these vital components of exercise prescription, we refer you back to Chapters 4–6.

When to Exercise

No one time of day is right for everyone. The right time for each patient will depend on her personal and professional schedule and preferences. If your patient is trying to manage weight by exercising, working out just before dinner may be preferable, as exercise promotes the secretion of insulin, the mobilization of glycogen (energy) from the liver, and the resultant suppression of hunger. Alternatively, the environment in which your patient lives may influence exercise patterns: in hot climates, exercise outside may be difficult during the middle of the day; while in cold climates, shorter days may prevent outdoor workouts after work. Some people like to start the day with a workout, either to get the day off to a "good start," often from the endorphins released while exercising, or to get their exercise "over with." Others feel that they are not yet fully awake, or do not have time in the morning, and would prefer to exercise at lunch or after work rather than before work. If your patient's workplace has changing facilities and showers, lunchtime workouts can be enjoyable and an effective use of time.

Sources of Reinforcement for Your Patient's New Habit

Even after exercising regularly for a short time, many patients start to "feel better" during or after exercising. At this early stage, your patient has likely not achieved many of the physiological gains of exercise, yet his *mind* has. Living in North America in this decade, your patient has undoubtedly heard about the benefits of exercise and knows that he "should" be more active. When he begins to succeed at committing to a program—even if the exercise amounts are below the recommended minimums—he will psychologically feel the benefits and the sense of accomplishment. Such emotions need to be encouraged, both by you and, if possible, by his family and friends. The physiological benefits will soon follow.

As your patient is preparing to start an exercise program, it is important for her to try to gain the support of family, friends, or employers. This support may come in the form of spouses offering to pick up the children to free up time for an after-work trip to the gym, a friend agreeing to get up for a morning walk each morning, or an employer offering incentives or facilities to encourage exercise. Although such external support is not mandatory for successful lifestyle change, it can be a great facilitator to becoming a regular exerciser.

Finally, as your patient's clinician, you have an important role to play in the success of his exercise program. Studies show that clinicians can be influential in the choices that their patients make (5–7). Through simple messages, the formal Exercise Prescription, and a show of genuine interest in your patient's progress, you can significantly impact the success of a patient's transition to an active lifestyle. Presenting tangible feedback regarding physiologic changes resulting from increased physical activity, *e.g.,* lowered blood lipids, decreased percentage of body fat, or improvement in blood pressure, is another form of support that clinicians can provide. By increasing your awareness and understanding of the process and importance of exercise prescription, you are already helping your patients move toward a healthier and more active lifestyle. We now challenge you to push, support, and encourage your patients to reach the ACSM/AHA recommendations.

The Exercise Environment: Where to Exercise?

One of the great things about becoming more active is that it can be done anywhere: from scheduled exercise outside, in the home, or in a fitness center; to small lifestyle changes that occur in a variety of environments, such as your commute, your stairs, your workplace—anywhere! This section focuses on three environments: outdoors, the home, and the gym or fitness center.

EXERCISING OUTDOORS

Perhaps the most common environment for exercising regularly is outdoors. Activities such as walking, jogging/running, cycling, golfing (walking the course and carrying the clubs), paddling, and gardening are most conducive to the outdoors. As with any environment, there are both advantages and disadvantages to exercising outside. Among the advantages are the ease and convenience of the outdoors. The convenience of being able to step out of one's home or office and immediately start walking, gardening, or jogging is appealing. As with any activity, task, or chore, the easier it is to do, the more likely it is to get done. In addition, many outdoor locations offer fresh air, variety, and sometimes beauty. Clearly, it is advisable for your patient to try to choose locations such as rural roads or parks in which to exercise. However, even within the heart of a city, nice places to exercise, such as parks, can often be found.

The main disadvantage of exercising outdoors is the potential safety risk. This risk can range from obstacles such as potholes in which your patient could sprain an ankle; to collisions with cars, dogs, or other people; to rare but dangerous situations with other people. Many of these risks can be mitigated though planning and common sense. Exercising at night, especially alone or in unlit areas, is not advisable. The safety section later in this chapter provides further tips for your patient to avoid risks such as those described here. In addition to the darkness, the weather can either help or hinder your patient's exercise plan. On warm sunny days, the desire to get outside may encourage your patient to walk, cycle, or garden; however, rain, snow, or extreme heat can have the opposite affect. Appropriate clothing, such as a water resistant but breathable jacket, sunscreen, or a belt to carry a water bottle can help your patient to overcome adverse weather conditions (see Chapter 12).

When exercising outdoors, the type of surface that your patient chooses to exercise on can impact both her enjoyment and her chance of injury. Exercising on the sidewalk or road provides your patient with an interesting trade-off. Sidewalks are generally safer, as they are farther from cars. However, a blacktop pavement offers significantly more resilience for your patient than a concrete sidewalk, and can therefore help prevent overuse injuries such as shin splints. If your patient chooses to exercise on lightly trafficked roads, she should walk or jog facing traffic. Parks often provide exercisers with dirt or grass paths on which to walk or run. While these paths are usually safer, (except at night), and more pleasant than roadways, patients should remain acutely aware of their surroundings—watching for both obstacles and dangerous situations. Just as a blacktop pavement is softer than cement, gravel or grass paths are softer than pavement.

Another potential outdoors exercise location is a local track. Many schools have tracks that are only used during certain hours or seasons. Tracks can provide a safe place to walk or run. For patients who are interested in finding out how fast they walk or run, timing themselves to complete four laps in the inside lane will give them their time per mile, as four laps of a standard track equal one mile. Because of the curve and gentle inward slope of most tracks, it is advisable to periodically change direction (*e.g.,* after every 4 laps) to prevent overuse injuries. Many busier tracks, however, may not allow this.

EXERCISING AT HOME

Many physical activities can easily be done at home. Some examples include using a stationary bike or treadmill, doing yoga or aerobics with a DVD or TV show, or resistance training (using dumbbells, household items such as soup cans, or lifting one's own body weight). The advantages of exercising at home are the safety, convenience, and comfort of one's own home. For parents with children, for example, it may be possible to exercise and "watch" the kids at the same time. There are, however, some potential disadvantages of exercising at home. Your patients may be easily distracted from their exercises by family members or other chores that need attention. Similarly, it is easy at home to procrastinate starting the workout by finding alternate tasks that take over your patient's exercise time.

EXERCISING AT A GYM OR FITNESS CENTER

Fitness centers, gyms, and "health clubs," by design, are great places to exercise. Some of the advantages of these facilities are the use of a wide variety of equipment for both cardiovascular and resistance training and the trained staff to assist your patient with their exercise program. Depending on your patient's medical precautions and the need for supervision, staff at the fitness center may be appropriate to monitor your patient's medical precautions. In addition, the music played at fitness centers and the ability to exercise in the presence of others who are also working hard to be healthy can be very motivating.

The primary disadvantage of exercising at a fitness center is the cost. Centers vary considerably in their prices and pricing packages. However, many clubs are available for around $500 per year. Patients who would like to exercise at a fitness center but have financial restrictions, should seek out different facilities such as community centers or YMCA/YMHAs. Other disadvantages can include the inconvenience of having to commute to the facility to exercise, hours of operation or of specific classes, and the possible intimidation of exercising with "all those fit people."

There are numerous factors that your patient should consider when choosing a fitness center. The first is location. If the center is not within 10–12 minutes from home or work, your patient will likely have a hard time motivating himself to go. Second, your patient should consider both the cleanliness and the atmosphere of the facility. Different types of centers will attract different types of individuals—from intense body builders to folks just there to "work out," the category that will likely include most of your patients. The type of people attending the gym can be either motivating or intimidating. "Women only" clubs, YMCAs, or community centers may provide a less intimidating environment for some patients.

Other environmental considerations include friendliness of staff and volume and type of music played. The facilities and classes offered by a fitness center may also influence your patient's decision to join and to continue going. Many offer a wide range of aerobic equipment (treadmills, stationary bikes, elliptical trainers, a swimming pool, etc.), machines designed for both cardiovascular and resistance training (stairmasters and rowing machines), resistance equipment (free weights or weight machines), and cardiovascular or resistance classes (aerobics, spin, yoga, pump, stepping, kick-boxing, etc.). Your patient will need to consider which of these factors are important for him, and weigh them against the cost of each facility. Some facilities have one price that allows members to use all facilities, while others offer different packages for different options.

Patients may choose one single environment in which to exercise, or they may combine or vary their choices. Some examples include walking briskly to the gym to attend a class or to use the weights for resistance training, going for a bike ride and then doing strengthening and stretching exercises at home, or focusing on running in the summer and swimming at a local pool in the winter.

SAFETY

Staying Alert and Defensive

Both for personal safety and to avoid injuries from collisions or obstacles, encourage your patients to stay alert and observant when exercising, especially outdoors. Cars and cyclists often have difficulty seeing pedestrians, necessitating a defensive approach by walkers, runners, rollerbladers, etc. Patients need to watch out not only for cars driving erratically on the roads, but also for cars turning or backing out of driveways, car doors opening, and other cyclists, pets, or pedestrians.

When on foot, patients should try to move against the flow of traffic so as to be able to see cars and react to them, but when passing others on a sidewalk or trail, should stay to the right and pass on the left, as is customary in a car. Cyclists, however, must by law move with traffic. Although exercising at night is not recommended, some patients may report that this is the only time that they can fit in a workout. Some tips to help these patients stay safe are to stick to well-lit routes, to exercise with a partner or a group, to wear flashing lights or a reflective vest or clothing, and, especially for women, to vary their routes.

Many exercisers report entering their "own little world" or "the zone" when focused on their activity, or when wearing headphones, which should never be worn while cycling outdoors. Although this feeling can be both enjoyable and relaxing, your patients should always maintain some level of awareness of their surroundings.

In some cases, it may be necessary for your patient to take advanced safety precautions. A whistle or bell can be useful for alerting cars or cyclists, and for scaring off both two and four-footed attackers. We do not recommend that your patients carry anything valuable, but do suggest that personal identification and information about any medical conditions or allergies is carried in case of an emergency.

When to Exercise: Safety Considerations

Different patients will have different preferences about when to exercise. There are, however, some safety considerations to bear in mind. Outdoor exercising at night is not recommended, especially in parks or on unlit roads. If your patient feels that her neighborhood is safe and well-lit, the following tips are advisable: stick to sidewalks, be particularly observant for external obstacles such as potholes or roots; and, especially if your patient is listening to music while exercising, ensure that she can still hear and is well aware of her surroundings.

Health

An important aspect of exercise safety is protecting oneself against injury and illness, primarily through preventive measures. As we explained in Chapter 3, there is a small but real risk of patients exacerbating (known or unknown) cardiac conditions through exercise. Therefore, patients should be aware of the symptoms of a cardiac event and should be advised to take these seriously. In particular, pain or strange feelings in the chest or arms that do not seem to be related to the specific muscles being exercised should be responded to quickly: your patient should stop the current exercise session and seek medical attention before returning to exercise.

More common and usually less serious are exercise-related injuries. These can be grouped into two classifications: intrinsic and extrinsic injuries. Intrinsic injury results from the activity itself—usually from exercising for too long, or too fast during a given session, or too much over a cumulative period of time. Thus, another term for intrinsic injury is "overuse injury." Examples include shin splints, swimmer's shoulder, tennis elbow, and a leg stress fracture. Also patients will commonly experience Delayed Onset Muscle Soreness (DOMS) in muscle groups that have not been active for months or longer. The increased demand on these muscles may result in somewhat severe pain in the several days after the new or increased level of activity. While there are no proven treatments for DOMS, patients often experience some relief with non-steroidal anti-inflammatory medications, gentle stretching, massage, or ice and heat. Extrinsic injuries result from collisions with an obstacle or other physical object: an automobile, a pothole, a dangling tree branch, another exerciser, or a strolling child and mother. The key to avoiding the first is simply not to do overdo it. The key to avoiding the second is, as noted above, to be aware of your surroundings, the road surface, traffic, and potential obstacles.

POTENTIAL OBSTACLES TO BECOMING (AND REMAINING) A REGULAR EXERCISER

As we highlighted in Chapter 6 (Behavior Change Pyramid), it is important for your patient to anticipate and thereby do her best to avoid potential roadblocks. Exercisers at all levels—from beginners to Olympians—face obstacles and setbacks. Accepting that obstacles will arise is an important first step to overcoming them. Events such as vacations, illness, or the arrival of house guests can alter your patient's regular routine, making exercising more difficult for a short period of time. Such breaks are not a problem, as long as your patient can return to exercising, potentially at a slightly lower level initially, after the interruption.

Motivational obstacles also occur in exercisers of all levels, but are often more common at the start of an exercise program. This is because beginner exercisers have not yet personally experienced the great benefits of exercising. At this early stage, encouragement and working through obstacles are necessary. If your patient is not enjoying the exercise, try to help him determine which component of the exercise is less enjoyable—is it the time of day? the frequency? the pace of the exercise? the type of exercise? Or is your patient frustrated that he has not yet seen the physical results of his hard work? Help your patient problem-solve through or around these obstacles, realizing that each patient's exercise program may need to be as unique as each patient. If you feel that you do not have the time or resources to address these concerns, be sure to refer your patient to a physical therapist or other exercise specialist for assistance.

Finally, your patient may complain that the exercise is causing pain or discomfort. One of the most common causes of pain is improper equipment (see Chapter 11). Ensure that your patient is using shoes that fit correctly and are designed for her foot type (over-pronation, neutral foot, or under-pronation). For walkers and runners, shoes should be changed every 350–550 miles to prevent injuries (8). At this stage, the shoes may not appear to be worn out, but their cushioning and stability will have deteriorated. Running stores, rather than generic sports stores, will be able to fit your patient into an appropriate walking, running, or aerobics shoe for a similar price to that of a generic sports store. Some muscle stiffness is common when increasing exercise. Such discomfort is not harmful so long as it does not last for more that a few days. In Chapter 11, we will provide further information on exercise equipment.

CONCLUSION

In this chapter, we have moved from the Foundation Phase of exercise (that included screening and motivating your patients) to the Becoming Active Phase, which we will discuss in more detail in the next chapter. In this phase, your patients actually start their physical activity. We have identified key principles to help your patients transform their lifestyle from sedentary to active, and have given you tips that you can use to help your patient find time to commit to exercise. We have also reviewed the different environments in which your patient can exercise, outlined potential safety concerns, and described potential obstacles that your patient may need to be aware of and to overcome.

In the following chapters, you will learn how to prescribe exercise to your patients in order to assist them in their transformation from a sedentary to an active lifestyle. In the process, you are given a choice. In Chapters 8 and 9, we will present general principles that should enable you to prescribe personalized exercise programs for your patients, based on their goals, health status, current fitness, and preferences. Alternatively, in Chapter 10, we offer you a specific pathway that takes your patient from a sedentary lifestyle to an active one, using a precise program. We recommend that you read all three chapters to understand the principles of exercise prescription, including important topics such as components of an exercise program, how to progress your patient, and how to prevent overtraining and injuries.

References

1. Haskell WH, Lee IM, Pate RR, Powell KE, Blair SN, Franklin BA, Macera CA. Physical activity and public health: updated recommendations for adults from the American College of Sports Medicine and the American Heart Association. Med Sci Sports Exer. 2007 August;39(8):1423–43.
2. American College of Sports Medicine. ACSM's guidelines for exercise testing and prescription. 8th ed. Philadelphia, PA: Lippincott Williams & Wilkins; 2009, pp. 152–182.

3. Pate RR, Pratt M, Blair SN, Haskell WL, Macera CA, Bouchard C, Buchner D. Physical activity and public health: a recommendation from the Centers for Disease Control and Prevention and the American College of Sports Medicine. JAMA. 1995 February;273(5):402–7.

4. U.S. Department of Health and Human Services, Centers for Disease Control. Physical activity and health: a report of the surgeon general. McLean (VA): International Medical Publishing; 1996. 278 p.

5. Redelmeier DA, Cialdini RB. Problems for clinical judgment: 5 principles of influence in medical practice Can Med Assoc J. 2002 June;166(13):1680–4.

6. Davis DA, Thomson MA, Oxman AD, Haynes RB. Changing physician performance: a systematic review of the effect of continuing medical education strategies. JAMA. 1995 September;274(9):700–5.

7. Cohen SJ, Stookey GK, Katz BP, Drook CA, Smith DM. Encouraging primary care physicians to help smokers quit. Ann Intern Med. 1989 April;110(8):648–52.

8. Pribut SM. Selecting a running shoe. Am Acad Pod Sports Med [Internet]. 2008 Feb [cited 2008 March 8]:[3 p.]. Available from: http://www.aapsm.org/selectingshoes.html

CHAPTER 8

The Exercise Prescription

Edward M. Phillips and Jennifer Capell

INTRODUCTION

You learned in Chapter 3 how to determine your patient's risk level and readiness for exercise. In Chapters 4, 5, and 6 you saw the importance of helping your patient lay the groundwork for regular physical activity through mobilizing motivation and developing a strategy for change, thereby beginning the move from Phase I—*Foundation* to Phase II—*Getting Active* (Figure 8.1). Now, you are ready to write the Exercise Prescription.

Chapters 3 and 4 discussed medical and mental assessment and screening of patients to determine their readiness to begin and/or maintain a program of regular physical activity. Patients in the Pre-Contemplative Stage—who are not yet ready, willing, and able to begin exercising—are advised of the benefits of exercise. At the other end of the spectrum, patients who already exercise can be counseled to maintain or to increase their exercise, as appropriate, and guided through a program to avoid injury, prevent relapse, and maintain interest in their exercise. Advice and counsel on regular exercise for this group is covered in Chapter 9. In this chapter, we focus on patients who are *contemplating* a program of regular exercise, or actively *planning* it. Depending on your type of clinical practice, you may have a significant number of patients who are starting to think seriously about becoming regular exercisers, but are still sedentary or minimally active. It is precisely on these patients, and their health, that your message to initiate and to maintain exercise will have the greatest effect. (See Figure 7.2.)

Just as in medical school students learn how to write prescriptions for medications, in this chapter you will learn how to write an exercise prescription. Although only certain health care professionals (*e.g.,* physicians, nurse practitioners, physicians' associates, and dentists) are licensed to prescribe medications, any clinician can legally write and provide exercise prescriptions to patients. We strongly recommend, however, that healthcare professionals without the legal authority to write medication prescriptions refer patients for a medical evaluation and possibly pre-exercise testing to determine if they have any significant health risks when attempting regular exercise (see Chapter 3).

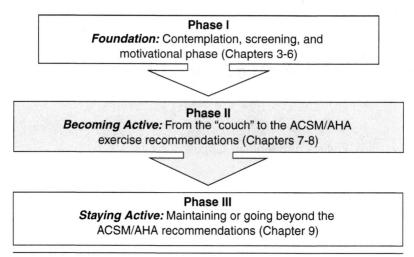

Figure 8.1 • The Phases of Lifestyle Change: From Sedentary to Active

When you have a patient who would benefit from a certain medication, it is your responsibility as a clinician to prescribe that medication, especially if *not* prescribing that medication would lead to disability, disease, or death. Given the proven health risks of a sedentary lifestyle (see Table 3.1), the Exercise is Medicine program is based on the concept that it is both the role and responsibility of a clinician to prescribe exercise to patients who would benefit from it. While even low levels of physical activity are better than inactivity, the prescribed program will hopefully guide the sedentary patient to achieve the national recommended levels. The first type of exercise prescription that we will cover is aerobic or cardiovascular exercise. We will then focus on resistance training as a separate type of exercise intervention, and then touch upon flexibility exercises. It is our hope that you will feel competent and even compelled to start writing simple, personalized exercise prescriptions for your patients by the time you finish reading and digesting the information presented in this chapter.

COMPONENTS OF THE EXERCISE PRESCRIPTION

The components of a prescription for medication include the name of the medication, strength or dose, frequency of administration, route, refills, and precautions. The components of an exercise prescription follow a similar format, using the FITT principle: **F**requency, **I**ntensity, **T**ime (or duration), and **T**ype. With a prescription medication, you may start a patient on a small dose and gradually increase the dosage to the full therapeutic level. Similarly, exercise prescription for a sedentary patient will begin at a minimal level, focusing first on the preliminary aspects of the regular exercise program. From this "small dose" of exercise, the patient, with your encouragement and guidance, will hopefully progress to at least the ACSM/AHA minimum recommended level of physical activity (1). Thus, in addition to the initial prescribed "dose" of exercise, the exercise *progression* is an important part of the prescription. We present three different pathways over which your patients can advance from a sedentary lifestyle to a regularly active lifestyle. First, let us define the different components of the exercise prescription.

Medication Prescription:

Medicine:	Ibuprofen
Strength:	600 mg tablets
Route:	By mouth
Dispense:	90 tablets
Frequency:	Three times per day
Precautions:	Discontinue for stomach upset
Refills:	3

Exercise Prescription:

Exercise:	Walk 30 minutes per day
Strength:	Moderate intensity
Frequency:	Five days per week
Precautions:	Increase duration of walking slowly to avoid injury
Refills:	Forever.

Frequency refers to the number of times the activity is performed each week. There is a positive dose–response relationship between the amount of exercise performed—as the amount (frequency and time or duration) of exercise performed increases, so do the benefits received. Therefore, the more a patient can exercise in a week, both in frequency and total time, the better the long-term outcomes will be for him. After a certain point, adding more exercise stops being beneficial, but this is not usually relevant for patients just beginning an exercise program, and will be discussed in Chapter 9.

Intensity of the physical activity is the level of vigor at which the activity is performed. There are a number of ways in which intensity can be measured. Some methods are easier to use but are generally less objective, while others are more objective but may require additional equipment or simple calculations. Table 8.1 provides an overview of some ways to measure exercise intensity.

In general, we recommend using a simple, though less objective, measure of intensity, such as the "talk test" or the Rating of Perceived Exertion (RPE). There may be situations in which you want to use or at least to understand the

TABLE 8.1 Measuring Exercise Intensity

| Intensity | Subjective Measures | | Physiological/ Relative Measures | | Absolute Measure |
	"Talk Test"	Perceived Exertion (10 point scale)	%HRR VO₂R (%)	Maximal HR (%)	METs VO₂max
Light	Able to talk and/or sing	< 3	< 40	< 64	< 3
Moderate	Able to talk but not sing	3–4	40–60	64–76	3–6
Vigorous/ hard	Difficulty talking	≥ 5	> 60	> 76	> 6

Abbreviations: METs = metabolic equivalent units (1 MET = 3.5 mL×kg^{-1}×min^{-1});
$\dot{V}O_2R$ = oxygen uptake reserve; HRR = heart rate reserve
Note: see Chapter 8 addendum for details on how to calculate measures of intensity
The "absolute measure" column is illustrative of a patient with a maximal aerobic capacity of around 8 METs.
From ACSM's Guidelines for Exercise Testing and Prescription. 8th ed. Philadelphia (PA): Lippincott Williams & Wilkins 2009, pp 152–182.

more objective measures. For a detailed explanation of these measures, please see the Guidelines for Exercise Testing and Prescription. In this section, we provide an overview of the more common methods; in the addendum to this chapter, we will review the calculation of percent of maximum heart rate (%HR$_{max}$), percent of heart rate reserve (%HRR), percent of oxygen consumption reserve (VO₂R), and metabolic equivalents (METS) (see definition in "absolute measures of intensity").

Subjective Measures of Intensity

The least objective but easiest measure of intensity is the "talk test." When performing physical activity at a low intensity, an individual should be able to talk or sing while exercising. At a moderate intensity, talking is comfortable, but singing, which requires a longer breath, becomes more difficult. At vigorous intensity, neither singing nor prolonged talking is possible (2). A similarly easy but more robust measure of intensity is "perceived exertion." The original perceived exertion scale, the Borg Rate of Perceived Exertion (RPE) Scale ran from a minimum of 6 to a maximum of 20. This scale has been simplified to a 10-point scale in which intensity increases from a minimum (level 0) to a maximum (level 10) (3). We generally recommend using the 10-point RPE scale for patients without significant cardiovascular risk factors.

Physiological/Relative Measures of Intensity

Other more objective measures include percentages of maximal oxygen consumption ($\dot{V}O2max$), oxygen consumption reserve ($\dot{V}O2R$), heart rate reserve (HRR), and maximal heart rate (HR_{max}). Some of these more objective measures are used in formal exercise testing. Perhaps the easiest but not the most accurate measure is calculated using a percentage of the patient's HR_{max}. For example, exercising at a moderate intensity would be quantified as 64%–75% of HR_{max} (4). You determine your patient's HR_{max} using the formula 220 minus the patient's age (220 − age). Although this method is simple, it has a high degree of variability and tends to underestimate HR_{max} in patients under the age of 40 and overestimate it in patients over the age of 40. This is generally true for both genders (4). A more accurate but more complicated formula is 206.9 − (0.67 × age) (5). Depending on the situation, the clinician will need to decide whether ease or accuracy is more important. Table 8.2 provides the projected heart rates at different ages and different intensities (using the HR_{max} formula 206.9 − (0.67 × age)).

Absolute Measures of Intensity

Metabolic equivalents (METs) represent the absolute expenditure of energy needed to accomplish a given task such as walking up two flights of stairs. One MET approximates the body's energy requirements at complete rest. METs are a useful and convenient way to describe the intensity of a variety of physical activities and are helpful in describing the work of different tasks; however, the intensity of the exercise needed to achieve that task is relative to the individual's reserve (6). For example, a healthy, active patient may report that climbing the two flights of stairs as light-intensity, while an inactive, chronically ill patient may report that the same task requires vigorous effort. Table 8.3 demonstrates the energy expenditure to perform different tasks.

In the joint American College of Sports Medicine (ACSM) and American Heart Association (AHA) exercise recommendations, light physical activity is defined as requiring less than 3 METs, moderate activities 3–6 METs, and vigorous activities greater than 6 METs (1).

As with other aspects of this book, you and the patient are offered choices. Here, again, which measure of intensity is used is up to the patient and you. For patients at risk for cardiac events, more objective measures may be necessary; while for otherwise healthy, sedentary patients, the easier, more subjective measures will likely suffice. (Refer to Table 8.1 for intensity measures.)

Time, or duration of the activity, refers to the length of time that the activity is performed. Generally, bouts of exercise that last for at least 10 minutes are added together to give a total time or duration for a given day (1). For example, a patient who walks 10 minutes to work, and 10 minutes back home, can count a total time or duration of 20 minutes for the day. Note that the exercise recommendations are dosed in terms of minutes of activity.

TABLE 8.2 Heart Rate Ranges for Low-, Moderate-, and Vigorous-Intensity Exercise (4)

Age	Low Intensity	Moderate Intensity	Vigorous Intensity	HR$_{max}$
15	< 126	126–150	> 150	197
20	< 124	124–147	> 147	194
25	< 122	122–145	> 145	190
30	< 120	120–142	> 142	187
35	< 117	117–139	> 139	183
40	< 115	115–137	> 137	180
45	< 113	113–134	> 134	177
50	< 111	111–132	> 132	173
55	< 109	109–129	> 129	170
60	< 107	107–127	> 127	167
65	< 105	105–124	> 124	163
70	< 102	102–122	> 122	160
75	< 100	100–119	> 119	157
80	< 98	98–117	> 117	153
85	< 96	96–114	> 114	150
95	< 92	92–109	> 109	143

Note: these ranges were calculated using the formula:

$[206.9 - (0.67 \times age)] \times \%HR_{max}$

Low intensity: <64% HR$_{max}$

Moderate intensity: 64%–76% HR$_{max}$

Vigorous intensity: >76% HR$_{max}$

Type of physical activity: Walking is the most common form of physical activity that sedentary individuals can begin. Walking is a very familiar activity, and one that can easily be incorporated into daily life. However, as Table 8.3 illustrates, there are a wide variety of other activities that your patient can choose.

As will be discussed further in Chapters 9 and 10, it is recommended that patients choose more than one activity that they enjoy to provide variety, to utilize different muscles, and to help prevent overuse injuries (7, 8). When discussing the exercise prescription with your patient, assist her in identifying activities that she is willing to pursue.

TABLE 8.3 Examples of Types of Physical Activity (with Associated Intensity in METs)

Light < 3 METs	Moderate 3–6 METs	Vigorous > 6 METs
Walking	**Walking**	**Walking, jogging & running**
Walking slowly around home, store or office = 2.0*	Walking 3.0 mph = 3.3*	Walking at very, very brisk pace (4.5 mph) = 6.3*
	Walking at very brisk pace (4 mph) = 5.0*	Walking/hiking at moderate pace and grade with no or light pack (<10 pounds) = 7.0
Household & occupation	**Household & occupation**	Hiking at steep grades and pack 10–42 pounds = 7.5–9.0
Sitting—using computer; work at desk using light hand tools = 1.5	Cleaning–heavy: washing windows, car, clean garage = 3.0	Jogging at 5 mph = 8.0*
	Sweeping floors or carpet, vacuuming, mopping = 3.0–3.5	Jogging at 6 mph = 10.0*
	Carpentry–general = 3.6	Running at 7 mph = 11.5*
Standing—performing light work such as making bed, washing dishes, ironing, preparing food or store clerk = 2.0–2.5	Carrying & stacking wood = 5.5	**Household & occupation**
	Mowing lawn–walk power mower = 5.5	Shoveling sand, coal, etc. = 7.0
		Carrying heavy loads such as bricks = 7.5
Leisure time & sports	**Leisure time & sports**	Heavy farming such as bailing hay = 8.0
Arts & crafts, playing cards = 1.5	Badminton–recreational = 4.5	Shoveling, digging ditches = 8.5
Billiards = 2.5	Basketball–shooting around = 4.5	**Leisure time & sports**
Boating–power = 2.5	Bicycling–on flat: light effort (10–12 mph) = 6.0	Basketball game = 8.0
Croquet = 2.5	Dancing–ballroom slow = 3.0; ballroom fast = 4.5	Bicycling–on flat: moderate effort (12–14 mph) = 8.0; fast (14–16 mph) = 10
Darts = 2.5	Fishing from river bank & walking = 4.0	Skiing cross country–slow (2.5 mph) = 7.0; fast (5.0–7.9 mph) = 9.0
Fishing–sitting = 2.5	Golf–walking pulling clubs = 4.3	Soccer–casual = 7.0; competitive = 10.0
Playing most musical instruments = 2.0–2.5	Sailing boat, wind surfing = 3.0	Swimming–moderate/hard = 8–11†
	Swimming leisurely = 6.0†	Tennis singles = 8.0
	Table tennis = 4.0	Volleyball–competitive at gym or beach = 8.0
	Tennis doubles = 5.0	
	Volleyball–noncompetitive = 3.0–4.0	

* On flat, hard surface. †MET values can vary substantially from person to person during swimming as a result of different strokes and skill levels.

Adapted from (1): Table 1.1 MET Values of Common Physical Activities Classified as Light, Moderate or Vigorous Intensity (Data from Ainsworth B, Haskell WL, White MC, et al. Compendium of physical activities: an update of activity codes and MET intensities. Med Sci Sports Exerc. 2000 September;32(9suppl):S498-S504).

In summary, the factors to keep in mind when prescribing exercise to your patient are the frequency, intensity, time (duration), and the type(s) of activity. These components can be remembered through the acronym FITT.

Although much of the focus for your patient's exercise program will be on the cardiovascular (aerobic) component, the ACSM/AHA guidelines also recommend patients include a resistance training component. In addition, there are a number of other components that you and/or your patient may consider. These include flexibility, and particularly for older patients, neuromuscular training (1). These topics will be addressed later in this chapter.

Now let's move on to the actual process of prescribing exercise to your sedentary patient.

WHERE TO BEGIN

Once you have determined that it is safe for your patient to begin exercising (see Chapter 3), that he is in the Contemplative or Planning Stage (see Chapter 4), and that he has undertaken the necessary motivational groundwork (Chapters 5 and 6), it is time to work with him to personalize an exercise program. The regular habit of exercise has been stressed as a critical component of adherence. It is now time to assist your patient in deciding which type of exercise he would like to do. As mentioned previously, walking is often the least intimidating and easiest to work into a patient's schedule; however, other exercises can and should be encouraged. Remember that patients who have been assessed to have a moderate level of risk should begin with low- or moderate-intensity exercises (see Table 8.3 for ideas).

Once your patient has identified the type(s) of exercise with which he is most comfortable, discuss with him the duration (amount of time per day) that he feels confident committing to exercising. He should be able to commit to this duration on at least three days each week. There are a number of components to this discussion that need to be elaborated on. First, your patient should begin exercising at a low- or moderate-intensity. For example, if your patient chooses to begin with a walking program, the walking can begin at a pace that is comfortable for the patient. The goal of this is to take the intimidation out of exercising. Reassure your patient that exercising does not have to involve intense activities such as running or playing competitive sports.

Second, ask your patient to consider a 10-point confidence scale, in which 1 is "not at all confident" and 10 is "100% sure she can do it," and to identify a length of time (*e.g.,* 5 minutes, 10 minutes, or 20 minutes) that she can commit to. She should have a confidence score of ≥ 7 out of 10.

Finally, we suggest that your patient commit to exercising at least three times per week. This recommendation stems from the observation that the hard part of "regular exercise" is the *regular,* not the *exercise* (see Chapter 7).

By strongly encouraging your patient to commit to at least three times per week, you can help him establish exercise as a regular "habit" in his life. If your patient is not confident that the duration goal that he set can be maintained at a frequency of at least three times each week, ask him to reconsider his duration goal, and to shorten it to an amount of time that he is confident he can maintain regularly (≥ 3 times/week). Once the starting duration has been determined, ask your patient to exercise at this level for 2–3 weeks before progressing his exercise program.

CASE STUDY

James is a 54-year-old male patient whom you have assessed to be at a moderate risk level (because of his age and sedentary lifestyle). It is safe for him to begin exercising at a low or moderate level, and he has demonstrated his readiness to pursue a simple exercise program. He does not feel that he has time to exercise, but is worried about his steady weight gain. He has decided that walking is the most realistic type of exercise for him to start with. James and his clinician discuss his exercise prescription:

CLINICIAN: *James, I am so glad that you are ready to begin making yourself healthier through physical activity. I think that a good way for you to get started is to commit to walking around the block for at least 20 minutes a day three days a week. The eventual goal will be to work up to 30 minutes of moderate-intensity walking at least five days a week. But, remember, we're going to start with the "regular," and worry about the "exercise" part later. Can you commit to walking at least 20 minutes per day at least three days per week as a start?*

JAMES: *Well, maybe, but I am really busy at work.*

CLINICIAN: *OK. How about starting out at 15 minutes each time, but on a regular schedule? On a scale of 1 to 10, how confident are you that you can do this three times per week?*

JAMES: *That seems more realistic. I will walk Saturday, Sunday, and Wednesday. I am 8-out-of-10 confident that I can do this.*

CLINICIAN: *Great, James. Let's start there. To begin with, walk at a pace that is comfortable for you. Over time, you will be walking at a brisker pace. Record on this log how many times you walk in the week and try to make sure that you get at least three walks in, each 15 minutes long, for two weeks. If that works for you, think about going to 20 minutes per time, three times per week. I look forward to seeing your log on your next visit in three weeks.*

It is permissible and often advisable to negotiate the details of the initial exercise prescription with your patient. This process will lead to both a realistic assessment of where your patient is in the motivational process and will provide an achievable initial goal.

PROGRESSION TO ACHIEVING THE ACSM RECOMMENDATIONS

Before you send your patient off to start her exercise program, the two of you will want to consider how and when she will progress her exercise program. It is assumed that your patient will eventually set a goal to reach the ACSM/AHA recommended levels of 150 minutes a week of moderate-intensity exercise or 60 minutes a week of vigorous-intensity exercise, or some combination thereof. She might do this at the outset, or she might do it only after conquering the "regular." It is important to remember that some patients will need some time to adjust to the changes in their lifestyle, and to convince themselves that they can and will benefit from a more active lifestyle. A balance will be needed between giving your patient time to adjust and encouraging her to challenge herself to attain her goals.

This progression can occur by increasing the duration, the frequency, the intensity, or a combination of these. There is no single correct order to progress these components, and the best option will vary depending on each patient's preferences, health status, and lifestyle. We will describe three different paths that your patients can choose to follow, each focusing on a different component: duration, frequency, and intensity. In each case, it is assumed that your patient is beginning his program for a duration that he is confident that he can maintain at least 3 times per week (frequency) at a low- to moderate-intensity (refer to Table 8.1 for ways to quantify levels of intensity).

The ACSM recommends that in order "to promote and maintain health, all healthy adults ages 18–65 yrs need:
- moderate-intensity aerobic activity for a minimum of 30 min on five days each week
- or vigorous-intensity aerobic activity for a minimum of 20 min on three days each week
- [or a combination] of moderate- and vigorous-intensity activity . . . to meet this recommendation" (1).

The Duration Path

This option allows your patient to continue exercising only three days each week, while increasing the duration of the exercise by 5–10 minutes every week (or less if she is older or is beginning at a very sedentary level). As she becomes more comfortable with the program, the intensity of the exercise, such as walking, can increase until she is at a moderate intensity as measured by a perceived exertion (RPE) level of 3–4 out of 10. She should be able to talk, but not sing during the exercise. This path enables your patient to more easily observe

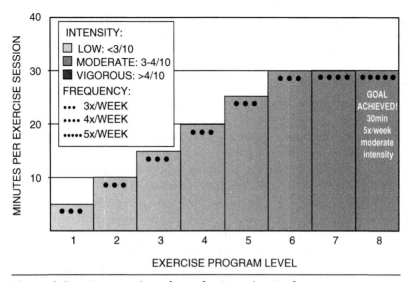

Figure 8.2 • Progression along the Duration Path

changes in fitness. For example, over a course of one month, she may go from walking five minutes a day three times each week up to 20 or even 30 minutes a day three times each week. Once a duration of 30 minutes is reached, your patient can then increase the frequency of the exercise from three times each week (in Figure 8.2 this occurs at the end of level 6), to four, and then five times each week. At this point, your patient should be congratulated for reaching the ACSM recommended exercise levels. Figure 8.2 illustrates this progression. If you and your patient determine that this is the most appropriate path of progression, use Patient Handout 8.1.

Let us return to James, the patient introduced above. Since he feels that he is pressed for time, he does not want to move up to exercising five days a week. Further, given his risk level, he should not increase to vigorous-intensity exercise until he has had his risk level reassessed. Therefore, the most appropriate progression plan for James is the duration path. He had committed to his physician to begin walking for 15 minutes three times a week. His clinician asked him to increase each session by 5 minutes every week. Together they discussed times in the day in which he could "slip in" exercise: a walk down to a coffee shop a block away instead of the one in his building; an extra block added onto his walk home; and then once he was up to 30 minutes a day, walking to and from work. Starting from 15 minutes three times each week, it took James five weeks to reach 30 minutes three times each week. It was particularly cold one week, so he lapsed back into taking the bus the whole way home from work that week. By the time he reached this point, he was actually enjoying his exercise and the extra energy he felt throughout the day. Having reached his first milestone of 30 minutes a day three days a week, James decided to start biking slowly to and from work twice a week, thereby increasing his exercise frequency to five days a week.

The Frequency Path

As an alternative to focusing the progression on duration of each exercise session, your patient can begin their progression by first increasing the frequency of activity up to at least five days each week, while maintaining the same duration for each session. Some patients will be able to increase their frequency directly from three to five times per week; others will want to progress more slowly—first, to four times per week, and then up to five. This option has the advantage of helping your patient establish a more regular habit of incorporating exercise into his daily routine. As we have stated again and again, the hardest part of regular exercise is the *regular,* not the exercise.

Following this progression pathway focusing on frequency, your patient establishes the pattern of regular exercise for a duration that is not intimidating or overwhelming. Once your patient has reached a frequency of at least five times each week, he can then consider increasing the intensity of the exercise to a moderate level, *i.e.,* an RPE of 3–4 out of 10, or a level at which he is able to talk but not sing. Your patient can also consider increasing the duration of the exercise sessions by 5–10 minutes per week, while still maintaining the good habit of exercising five days each week. The order in which the intensity and duration are increased is not important and will depend on your patient's preference and health/fitness/age status. It is important that the patient is motivated to continue working towards the goal of reaching the ACSM/AHA recommendations. As with the duration path, once your patient has reached the target of 30 minutes of moderate intensity exercise at least five times each week, he should be congratulated. Figure 8.3 and the associated Patient Handout 8.2 illustrate this progression path.

We can explore the frequency progression through another patient vignette: Margaret is a 43-year-old woman with a blood pressure of 160/100. She smokes and is very sedentary. Lately, she has been feeling somewhat depressed. On a previous visit, her clinician began discussing the idea of becoming a little more active. At the time, she did not respond. On subsequent visits, she asked questions that indicated to her clinician that she had been contemplating becoming more active, but felt it was an overwhelming idea. She was assessed at a moderate risk level for exercise due to her blood pressure, smoking, and inactivity. After discussions around motivation, benefits, and barriers to becoming more active, Margaret committed to walking around the block (5 minutes) in the morning and the evening, three times a week. Although her clinician usually likes patients to begin with at least 10 minutes of continuous exercise, she thought that in Margaret's case, this was a good starting point, as "something is better than nothing" and because Margaret was so apprehen-

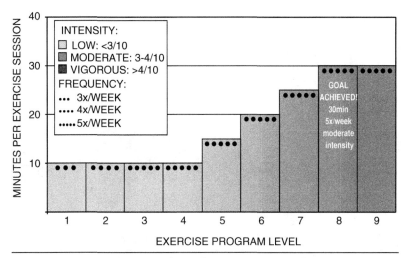

Figure 8.3 • Progression along the Frequency Path

sive about the idea of becoming more active. Note the use of the less intimidating phrase "more active" rather than "exercising" with Margaret, even though they are essentially the same thing. Margaret did not feel that she was ready to "exercise" but was willing to try being "just a bit more active."

Since Margaret was comfortable with the first few weeks of walking around the block, she and her clinician decided that when Margaret was ready to progress, she would increase the frequency of her walks to daily, rather than increasing the duration. Given Margaret's very sedentary baseline, her progression was set to increase every two weeks rather than weekly.

She first progressed to four times each week, and then to five. She was still walking fairly slowly at low intensity, but her clinician was pleased with her progress and encouraged her frequently. After almost two months, Margaret was ready to lengthen her morning walk to 10 minutes (keeping her evening walk at five minutes). She slowly continued with her daily exercise, gradually increasing the duration and then eventually the speed at which she was walking. She had come to know some of the neighbors through her regular walks, and began to look forward to the social interactions during her walks. Over a period of six months, Margaret managed to get herself into the minority of the US population who are physically active at the recommended levels. She now walks for 15 minutes in the morning and in the evening, five days a week. Her pace is not fast, but is at a level that she considers an intensity of 3–4 out of 10.

As part of the positive benefits of Margaret becoming "just a bit more active," she was pleased to get feedback from her physician. As a result of her physical activity, her blood pressure has decreased several points, her blood lipids improved, and her resting heart rate has reduced. She feels less depressed and more in control of her life.

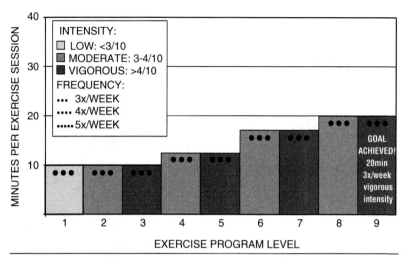

Figure 8.4 • Progression along the Intensity Path

The Intensity Path

The previous two progression paths assume that either your patient does not want to increase the intensity of his exercise (*e.g.,* from a walking program to a running program) or that his health condition prohibits this increased intensity. Remembering back to the pre-exercise assessment in Chapter 3, it is safe for patients at a moderate risk level (for example, those with ≥2 cardiovascular risk factors) to begin exercising at a moderate intensity, but they should obtain further medical evaluation and possible testing prior to exercising at a vigorous intensity. This third progression path will lead patients to the ACSM/AHA goal for vigorous intensity exercise. This path is designed for patients with low cardiovascular risk, especially those who want to exercise more vigorously, or who feel that they do not have time to exercise 150 minutes every week. The ACSM minimum weekly exercise recommendations for vigorous exercise, such as jogging, suggest that patients should exercise at least 20 minutes three times per week for a total of at least 60 minutes each week. The progression to this target/threshold is depicted in Figure 8.4 and Patient Handout 8.3.

To begin this progression, patients should first increase the intensity and duration of their exercise to at least a brisk 20-minute walk, three times per week. From this point, a walk-run program can be initiated. Each session should begin with a 5-minute brisk walk to warm up, followed by cycles of brisk walking and running. For example, in the first week, the cycle would consist of 1 minute of running followed by 1.5 minutes of walking. This can then be repeated six times (including the 5-minute warm-up, the total exercise time will be 20 minutes). The patient can continue to progress through the run-walk cycles outlined in Table 8.4. It is important to remind your patients to

TABLE 8.4 Progressing from Walking to Jogging—
3 times/week Program

Week	Run Time in Minutes	Walk Time in Minutes	Number of Times to Repeat Cycle	Total Exercise Time (excluding 5 min warm-up)	Comments
1	1	1.5	6	15 min	Begin each session with a 5-min brisk walk
2	1.5	2	4–5	14–16 min	
3	2	2	4	16 min	
4	3	3	3	18 min	The walk "breaks" between the run times should also be **brisk** walks
5	3	2	3–4	15–20 min	
6	3	1	4	16 min	
7	5	2	2	14 min	
8	8	2	2	20 min	
9	9	1	2	20 min	Some patients may choose to stay at this level (9:1 ratio) indefinitely, either maintaining a 20 min duration, or gradually increasing the total duration beyond the recommended activity levels.
10	1st run 12 2nd run 5	1	1	18 min	First run is 12 min, followed by a 1-min walk then a second run of 5 min
11	15	0	1	15 min	
12	17	0	1	17 min	
13	20	0	1	20 min	Warm up can be slower jog (instead of the brisk walk)

maintain a brisk walk during the "rest" periods. By doing so, your patient will maintain her increased heart rate, thus gaining physiological benefit from both the run and the walk time.

Some patients may chose to move through this walk-run program as a progression after taking the duration or frequency paths, thus giving more time to build up exercise endurance. Others may choose to continue to progress their walk-run or run program beyond the ACSM/AHA minimum recommendations. The recommendations support pursuing exercise beyond these minimum recommendations: "Because of the dose-response relationship between physical activity and health, persons who wish to further improve their personal fitness, reduce their risk for chronic diseases and disabilities, or prevent unhealthy weight gain may benefit by exceeding the minimum recommended amounts of physical activity" (1).

Chapter 9 will cover regular exercise progressions beyond these minimum recommendations. Although a patient may initially be assessed to have ≥2 cardiovascular risk factors and therefore be advised not to pursue vigorous exercise, he may in fact lower his risk through a regular, moderate-intensity exercise program. In this way, a patient who is initially at a moderate risk level can progress to vigorous exercise over time. The following vignette illustrates this.

Remember our patient James, the 54-year-old male who began a walking program and then progressed to walking and bicycle riding? He began his program at a moderate risk level due to his age and his sedentary lifestyle. About three 3 months after he began his exercise program, he was promoted at work and feared that he was not going to have time for the 150 minutes of exercise that he had been getting. He had to decrease his exercising back down to 60 minutes (walking briskly about 20 minutes three times a week) due to lack of time. He was disappointed since he was enjoying the exercise, so he returned to his clinician to discuss the issue. He had his exercise risk level reassessed; his age still acted as a risk factor. Since he was no longer inactive, the sedentary risk factor was removed, moving him up into the low risk category. Feeling quite proud of himself and the impact the exercise was having on his health, he began a walk–run program as described above. Over a period of 12 weeks, he had transformed his 60 minutes of walking to 60 minutes of jogging (vigorous intensity exercise), meeting the ACSM exercise recommendations.

Figure 8.5 provides a summary of the three progression paths from which your patient, with your assistance, can choose. Once a path has been chosen, you can give your patient a prescription corresponding to her path (see addendum 2 for prescription "pads"). This prescription should be personalized to her goal, starting level, and rate of progression. In addition to the ACSM/AHA recommendations for aerobic (cardiovascular) training, patients should also engage in resistance or strength training on a regular basis. We will now turn our attention to the prescription of resistance training exercises.

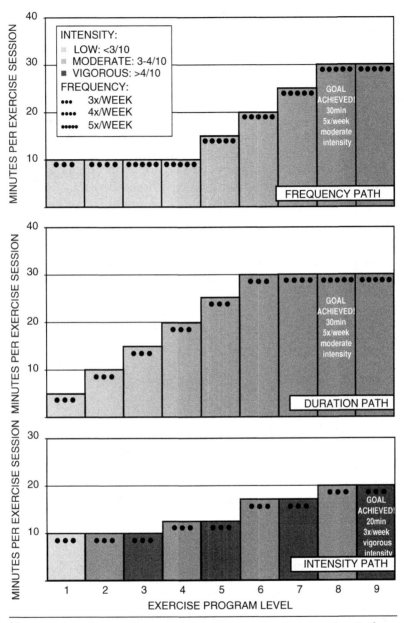

Figure 8.5 • Comparison of the Three Exercise Progression Paths

RESISTANCE (STRENGTH) TRAINING

In addition to the recommendations for aerobic activity, the ACSM suggests that in order "to promote and maintain good health and physical independence, adults will benefit from performing activities that maintain or increase muscular strength and endurance for a minimum of two days each week. It is recommended that 8–10 exercises be performed on two or more nonconsecutive days each week using the major muscle groups" (1). As summarized in Table 8.5, the benefits of Resistance (strength) training are numerous.

For most of your patients, you will prescribe resistance training to complement your patients' cardiovascular training. Follow the same FITT format:

Frequency: The ACSM/AHA recommends that patients participate in strengthening exercises on at least two non-consecutive days each week.

Intensity: The amount of resistance used should be heavy enough that your patient is able to complete only 8–12 repetitions before needing a break. The patient should be able to complete three sets of 8–12 repetitions with short (1–4 minutes) breaks in between each set.

Time (duration): Resistance training sessions do not need to consume a large amount of time—a routine consisting of three sets of 8–12 repetitions for 8–10 different muscle groups should take about 30 minutes.

Type: As with cardiovascular training, there is a wide variety of resistance exercises that patients can participate in. The most common types are strength training using weights such as dumb bells, bars, or weight machines found in gyms. Resistance training can also be done at home, using body weight, elastic cords, or even household objects such as soup cans. Alternative types of muscle-strengthening activities include stair-climbing, weight bearing calisthenics, and other resistance exercises that use the major muscle groups (2). Strengthening for general conditioning should focus on the major muscle groups of the arms (biceps, triceps, and

---

TABLE 8.5 Benefits of Resistance (Strength) Training (9)

- Reduces pain and disability associated with arthritis
- Restores balance and reduction of falls
- Strengthens bone
- Maintains proper weight
- Improves glucose control and consequently diabetes control
- Maintains a healthy state of mind and reduces symptoms of depression
- Improves sleep
- Improves heart muscle functioning

TABLE 8.6 Resistance Training: Principles and Prescription

Principles (10)

- Use both concentric and eccentric muscle actions
- Perform both single- and multiple-joint exercises
- Sequence exercises to optimize the quality of the exercise intensity (large before small muscle group exercises, multiple-joint exercises before single-joint exercises, and higher intensity before lower intensity exercises)

Sample Resistance Exercises for Major Muscle Groups

Instructions to patient (10):

- Do each of the following exercises 8–12 times (repetitions) and then rest for 1–2 minutes
- Repeat this two more time for a total of three sets
- Use a resistance (weight) that allows you to complete the 8–12 repetitions, but to feel fatigued at the end of each set

Exercises (11):

1. Dumbbell press—pectoral muscles (front of chest)
2. 'Bent over' row with dumbbell—shoulders and upper back
3. Arm curl with dumbbell—biceps
4. Elbow extension—triceps
5. Seated knee extension (with ankle weight)—quadriceps
6. Leg press—quadriceps, hamstrings, and gluteal muscles in your buttocks.
7. Hamstring curls
8. Push-up—chest, arms shoulders and upper body
9. Calf raise—gastrocnemius and soleus
10. Squat—quadriceps and gluteal muscles

---

deltoids), legs (quadriceps, hamstrings, and calves), and core (lower abdominals and back). Table 8.6 provides an example of exercises for these major muscle groups.

Introducing Resistance Training

Commonly, even patients who are physically active and pursue the recommended dose of regular cardiovascular exercise do not perform resistance exercises. As a slow progression to avoid injury and muscle soreness, your patient should be advised to initiate the resistance exercises at a lower intensity (*e.g.,* a perceived exertion of 5 or 6 on a 10-point scale) and at a lower resistance, such that she may complete 15 repetitions before fatiguing. In the first week, only one set of each of the exercises is done on two non-consecutive days. During week 2, the exercises are repeated at the same intensity, but a second set is added. During week 3, the resistance is raised such that your patient can now only complete 8–12 repetitions before she fatigues. The perceived

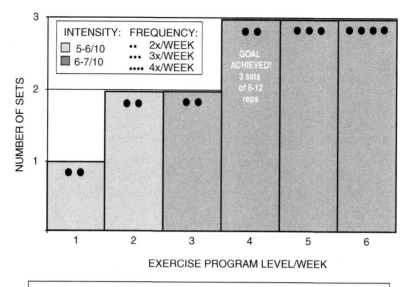

Figure 8.6 • Exercise Progression for Resistance Training

exertion of each set will now be 6 or 7 on a 10-point scale, or described as "really challenging."

Progression: As illustrated in Figure 8.6, in week 4 the third set of each resistance exercise is added. Your patient has now achieved the minimum ACSM/AHA recommendations for resistance training. Further progression may include additional sessions each week or slowly increasing the resistance such that the patient continues to reach a point of "really challenging" perceived exertion at the end of each set of exercises.

Adding a variety of resistance exercises is beneficial. If your patient is interested in increasing the type and variety of resistance training, it may be advisable to recommend that he seeks the assistance of a qualified health and fitness professional at a local fitness club for ideas on ways to add variety. Otherwise, maintaining a two-times-per-week program with progressively heavier weights will suffice.

FLEXIBILITY, BALANCE TRAINING, AND CORE STABILITY

Flexibility

There are also a number of other exercise components that your patient may wish to discuss with you. One such component is flexibility training. The research is not clear as to the benefit of warm-up exercises, therefore there are no specific recommendations. However, your patients may wish to go through the movements of the physical activity at the start and performing them at a slower pace than will be done during the 'main' exercise period. For example, the walk-run program described above begins each session with brisk walking. Stretching should be done once the muscles are warmed, either following the warm-up phase, or at the end of the exercise session. The patient should hold each stretch for 20–30 seconds and should feel a gentle tension, *not* pain. Although the benefits of stretching on acute athletic performance are still being debated, stretching is recommended to improve and to prevent the losses in range of motion that are associated with aging (4). The ACSM recommends that most adults include a stretching exercise program of at least 10 minutes in duration a minimum of two to three days each week. The stretches should include the major muscle groups of the body, with four or more repetitions per muscle group. Stretching exercises should be performed to the limits of comfort within the range of motion, but no further. This will be perceived as the point of mild tightness without discomfort (4).

Balance Training

Balance training is another important form of exercise. The ACSM/AHA recommendations that we refer to throughout the book are designed for adults under the age of 65. Especially for patients who are over this age, as well as for those who are severely deconditioned (7), simple exercises designed to improve balance are important. Such exercises include standing on one leg supported or unsupported, and with the eyes open or closed depending on your patient's ability, and walking in a straight line with one foot in front of the other. Specific guidelines and recommendations for older patients are discussed in Chapter 13. In addition the NIH website provides a series of balance exercises designed specifically for older adults (12).

Core Strengthening

In recent years, core stability training has emerged as an important component of physical fitness (13,14). The "core" is the central portion of the body: the trunk and its link to the extremities. Core stability refers to the ability to control the position and movement of the trunk in order to optimize movement and power in the extremities (13). Core stability exercises are designed to increase strength and endurance to the postural muscles of the trunk and pelvis, and are important for injury prevention and rehabilitation, particularly for low-back injuries. Performing exercises on an unstable surface such as a Swiss ball (Physioball) or a balance disc (wobble board); using free weights rather than machines; exercising one side at a time; and standing rather than sitting to perform exercises can help your patient to strengthen her core.[15]

CONCLUSION

In this chapter you have been guided through the process of actually writing an exercise prescription. The starting point and path of progression are negotiated with the patient. Similarly, the goal of moderate-intensity physical activity or shorter sessions of vigorous-intensity exercise have been determined by the patient's risk factors and his preference. Both cardiovascular and resistance training have been addressed. The national recommendations also indicate that greater amounts of exercise may confer greater benefits (1). In the next chapter we help you guide your patient to maintain these levels of activity, or to progress to more vigorous or longer-duration exercise. In Chapter 10, we will provide an alternative approach to exercise prescription. We will provide a specific program, called TSTEP, that you may prefer to prescribe to some patients.

APPENDIX: QUANTIFYING EXERCISE INTENSITY USING DIFFERENT METHODS

For those who are interested, the following section provides detailed information on calculating intensity using the following measures:

1. Percentage of maximal heart rate ($\%HR_{max}$)
2. Intensity percentage of heart rate reserve (HRR)
3. Oxygen consumption reserve ($\dot{V}O_2R$)
4. Metabolic equivalents (METS)

The calculations use the intensity ranges recommended by the ACSM's Guidelines for Exercise Testing and Prescription. 8th ed. Philadelphia (PA): Lippincott Williams & Wilkins 2009, pp 152–182 and are presented in Table 8.1 on page 102.

> The formula for calculating a target heart rate (THR) range using percent of maximal heart rate ($\%HR_{max}$) is: $THR = HR_{max} \times$ desired %

1. **Percentage of Maximal Heart Rate ($\%HR_{max}$)**

   In order to calculate a target heart rate (THR) based on a percentage of your patient's HR_{max}, you must first either know (from exercise testing) or calculate her HR_{max}. The simplest way to calculate HR_{max} is using the formula $HR_{max} = 220 -$ age; however, this method is not the most accurate (see discussion on page 103). A more accurate, but slightly more complicated method is the formula $HR_{max} = 206.9 - (0.67 \times$ age)

   Once the predicted HR_{max} for your patient is established, multiply this number by the percent of HR_{max} that you would like your patient to exercise at. For example, the ACSM suggests that moderate-intensity exercise should be performed at 64%–76% of HR_{max}.

   For example, if you would like your 51-year-old patient to exercise at moderate intensity, then the calculation would be as follows:

Data: 51-year-old patient

Moderate-intensity exercise = 64%–76% of HR_{max}

   Target Heart Rate **(THR) = $HR_{max} \times$ desired %**

Using **$HR_{max} = 220$-age**

   $HR_{max} = 220 - 51 = 169$

Lower range (64%) = $0.64 \times 169 = 108$

Upper range (76%) = $0.76 \times 169 = 128$

Using the $220 -$ age HR_{max} calculation, this patient should **exercise at a HR range of 108 to 128 beats per minute**

Using **$HR_{max} = 206.9 - (0.67 \times age)$**

   $HR_{max} = 206.9 - (0.67 \times 51) = 173$

Lower range (64%) = $0.64 \times 173 = 111$

Upper range (76%) = $0.76 \times 173 = 131$

Using the $206.9 - (0.67 \times age)$ HR_{max} calculation, this patient should **exercise at a HR range of 111 to 131 beats per minute**

2. **Intensity Percentage of Heart Rate Reserve (HRR)**

   Using heart rate reserve (HRR) is a more accurate measure of rate of energy expenditure and, therefore, exercise intensity. This method calculates the difference between a patient's maximal and resting heart rates, *i.e.,* heart rate reserve or "usable" heart rate range, and then multiplies this number by exercise intensity (percent). In order to use this method, the patient's resting and maximal heart rates need to be known or estimated using the calculations above.

   The formula for calculating a target heart rate (THR) range using heart rate reserve (HRR) is: $THR = [(HR_{max} - HR_{rest}) \times \% \text{ intensity}] + HR_{rest}$

   For example, suppose you are treating a patient who has a resting heart rate (HR_{rest}) of 64 beats per minute and a maximal heart rate (HR_{max}) of 189 beats per minute, and you would like him to exercise at a vigorous rate (>60% HRR), then in order to determine his target heart rate (THR), complete the following calculation.

   Data: HR_{rest}: 64 beats/min

   HR_{max}: 189 beats/min

   Exercise intensity: 60% of HRR

   [***Note:*** If your patient's HR_{max} is not known, you will need to begin by calculating a predicted HR_{max}. This is described in the above calculation ($\%HR_{max}$)]

   $$THR = [(HR_{max} - HR_{rest}) \times \% \text{ intensity}] + HR_{rest}$$
   $$= [(189 - 64) \times 0.6] + 64$$
   $$= [125 \times 0.6] + 64 = 139 \text{ beats per minute}$$

   Since you would like the patient to exercise at a rate greater than this 60% HRR, you would **suggest that he tries to keep his heart rate above (greater than) 139 beats/min.**

   In the above example, instead of using a heart rate range, it was recommended that the patient maintain a heart rate *above* an intensity of 60% HRR. If you had wanted him to maintain a heart rate within a range, *e.g.,* between 60% and 80% of HRR, then the 60% HRR calculation would become the lower limit of the range, and the calculation would need to be repeated for the 80% upper limit to the range, as shown in the previous example on $\%HR_{max}$.

3. **Oxygen Consumption Reserve ($\dot{V}O_2R$)**

   A very similar and equally accurate method of calculating rate of energy expenditure (intensity) to HRR is oxygen consumption reserve ($\dot{V}O_2R$). This similarity is because of the direct, linear relationship between these two measures of exercise intensity (8). The formulas used in the two calculations are the same, except that the resting and maximal heart rates in the HRR method is replaced with the patient's resting and maximal oxygen consumption ($\dot{V}O_{2rest}$ and $\dot{V}O_{2max}$). In practical terms, this change in the formula means that you need to know your patient's oxygen consumption, a variable that is generally more difficult because it requires more equipment to measure than heart rates.

The formula for calculating a target oxygen consumption (TVO_2) range using oxygen consumption reserve (VO_2R) is:

$$TVO_2 = [(\dot{V}O_{2max} - \dot{V}O_{2rest}) \times \% \text{ intensity}] + \dot{V}O_{2rest}$$

Note the similarity between this formula and the formula for HRR (above).

For example (adapted from ACSM's Guidelines for Exercise Testing and Prescription. 8th ed. Philadelphia (PA): Lippincott Williams & Wilkins 2009, pp 152–182, Figure 7.2), consider a patient who has a resting oxygen consumption ($\dot{V}O_{2rest}$) of 3.5 mL/kg/min and a maximal oxygen consumption ($\dot{V}O_{2max}$) of 30 mL/kg/min. You want to recommend that she exercises at a moderate intensity (40%–60% of VO_2R).

Data: $\dot{V}O_{2rest}$ = 3.5 mL/kg/min

$\dot{V}O_{2max}$ = 30 mL/kg/min

Exercise intensity = 40% to 60% of $\dot{V}O_2R$

Target VO_2 = [($\dot{V}O_{2max} - \dot{V}O_{2rest}$) × % intensity] + $\dot{V}O_{2rest}$

Lower limit of range (40%) = $[(30 - 3.5) \times 0.4] + 3.5 = 10.6 + 3.5 = 14.1$ mL/kg/min

Upper limit of range (60%) = $[(30 - 3.5) \times 0.6] + 3.5 = 15.9 + 3.5 = 19.4$ mL/kg/min

This patient should try to keep her oxygen consumption between 14.1 and 19.4 mL/kg/min.

4. **Metabolic Equivalents (METS)**

One metabolic equivalent is the measure of the amount of energy (oxygen) used by the body when sitting quietly (16), *i.e.,* the resting metabolic rate (RMR). When considering different forms of physical activity, METS express the energy cost of an activity as a multiple of the RMR (17). Numerically, one MET is equal to 3.5 mL/kg/min (4). Since these are the same units as used for VO_2, we can convert VO_2 measures into METS.

Given that 1 MET = 3.5 mL·kg^{-1}·min^{-1}, we can use cross multiplication to convert the VO_2 range to a METS range: **Desired MET = VO_2 / 3.5**

Let us continue with the VO_2R example from above. We determined that in order to exercise at a moderate intensity (40% to 60% of VO_2R), the patient should maintain her oxygen consumption (VO_2) between 14.1 and 19.4 mL/kg/min. We will now convert this VO_2 into METS.

Data: Lower limit of VO_2 range = 14.1 mL/kg/min

Upper limit of VO_2 range = 19.4 mL/kg/min

1 MET = 3.5 mL/kg/min (*Note:* this is always the case, not just in this example.)

Desired MET = VO_2 / 3.5

Lower MET target: 1 MET / 3.5 mL/kg/min = (× MET) / (14.1 mL/kg/min)

X MET = (14.1 mL/kg/min) / (3.5 mL/kg/min) = 4.0 MET

Upper MET target: 1 MET / 3.5 mL/kg/min = (× MET) / (19.4 mL/kg/min)

X MET = (19.4 mL/kg/min) / (3.5 mL/kg/min) = 5.5 MET

This patient should try to **engage in exercises that require an energy expenditure of between 4 and 5.5 METS.** Refer to Table 8.3 for examples of types of exercise and their METs.

Patient Handout 1: Exercise Prescription "Pad"–Duration Path

Exercise is Medicine   Clinician's Name: _____

Exercise Prescription for _____

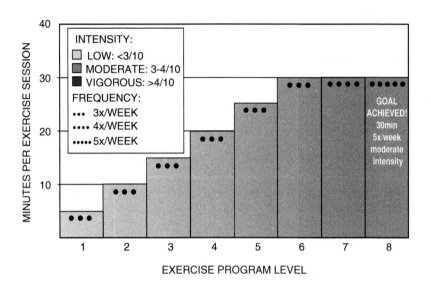

GOAL:

To _____ times each week for at least ____ minutes each time by
  (type of exercise) (#)   *(#)*

_____.
(target date)

In order to reach this goal, begin with the following:

BEGIN WITH:

Frequency   **F** _____ times each week

Intensity   **I** _____ intensity (*i.e.,* an intensity where you can <u>talk / sing</u>
                              while active)   *(circle)*

Time/duration **T** _____ minutes each day

Type   **T** _____ type of exercise (*e.g.,* walking, gardening,
                              swimming, etc.)

This corresponds to level _____ on the graph above.

Maintain this level for _____ weeks before starting your progression

PROGRESSION:

Every <u>week 1 / 2 weeks,</u> progress to the next level on the graph above.

     (circle)

PRECAUTIONS:

OTHER NOTES:

Patient Handout 2: Exercise Prescription "Pad"–Frequency Path

Exercise is Medicine   Clinician's Name: _____

Exercise Prescription for _____

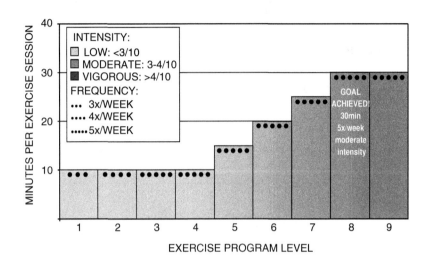

GOAL:

To _____ times each week for at least ___ minutes each time by
   (type of exercise) (#)   *(#)*

_____.
(target date)

In order to reach this goal, begin with the following:

BEGIN WITH:

Frequency   **F** _____ times each week

Intensity   **I** _____ intensity (*i.e.,* an intensity where you can <u>talk / sing</u>
                                    while active)   *(circle)*

Time/duration **T** _____ minutes each day

Type   **T** _____ type of exercise (*e.g.,* walking, gardening,
                                    swimming, etc.)

This corresponds to level _____ on the graph above.

Maintain this level for _____ weeks before starting your progression

PROGRESSION:

Every <u>week 1 / 2 weeks,</u> progress to the next level on the graph above.

       (circle)

PRECAUTIONS:

OTHER NOTES:

Patient Handout 3: Exercise Prescription "Pad"–Intensity Path

Exercise is Medicine

Clinician's Name: _____

Exercise Prescription for _____

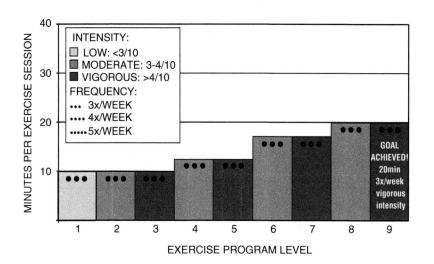

GOAL:

To _____ times each week for at least ___ minutes each time by

   (type of exercise) (#)   *(#)*

_____.

(target date)

In order to reach this goal, begin with the following:

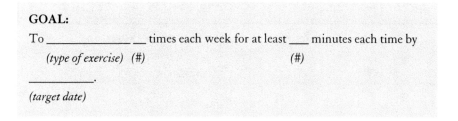

BEGIN WITH:

Frequency   **F** _____ times each week

Intensity   **I** _____ intensity (*i.e.,* an intensity where you can <u>talk / sing</u>
                                while active)   *(circle)*

Time/duration **T** _____ minutes each day

Type   **T** _____ type of exercise (*e.g.,* walking, gardening,
                                swimming, etc.)

This corresponds to level _____ on the graph above.

Maintain this level for _____ weeks before starting your progression

PROGRESSION:

Every <u>week 1 / 2 weeks,</u> progress to the next level on the graph above.

(circle)

PRECAUTIONS:

OTHER NOTES:

Patient Handout 4: Exercise Prescription for Resistance Training

Exercise is Medicine   Clinician's Name: _____

Exercise Prescription for _____

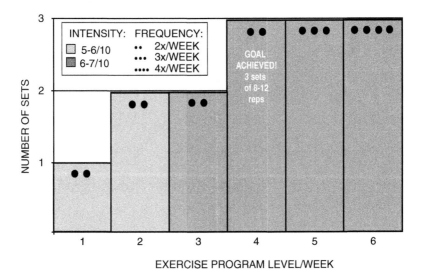

EXERCISE PROGRAM LEVEL/WEEK

In weeks 1 and 2 perform 15 repetitions until fatigue. In weeks 3 and beyond, increase resistance so that you can perform only 8-12 repetitions until fatigue.

GOAL:
To do resistance training two times each week for three sets of 8–12 repetitions in 8–10 different muscle groups.

In order to reach this goal, begin with the following:

BEGIN WITH:

Frequency   **F** _____ times each week

Intensity   **I** _____ intensity (*e.g.,* 3–4 on a 10-point scale of perceived exertion)

Time/duration **T** _____ one set each session.

Type   **T** _____ type of exercise (*e.g.,* lifting weights, resistance bands, etc.)

This corresponds to level _____ on the graph above.

PROGRESSION:

Every <u>week 1 / 2 weeks,</u> progress to the next level on the graph above.

    (circle)

PRECAUTIONS:

OTHER NOTES:

References

1. Haskell WH, Lee IM, Pate RR, Powell KE, Blair SN, Franklin BA, Macera CA, Heath GW, Thompson PD, Bauman A. Physical activity and public health: updated recommendations for adults from the American College of Sports Medicine and the American Heart Association. Circulation. 2007 Aug;116(9): 1081–93. [NOTE: this is referred to as Recommendations, 2007 in the text.]
2. Persinger R, Foster C, Gibson M, Fater DC, Porcari JP. Consistency of the talk test for exercise prescription. Med Sci Sports Exerc. 2004 Sep;36(7):1632–6.
3. Chen M, Fan X, Moe ST. Criterion-related validity of the Borg ratings of perceived exertion scale in healthy individuals: a meta-analysis. J Sports Sci 2002 Nov; 20(11):873–900.
4. Garber ME. Exercise prescription. In: American College of Sports Medicine, ed. ACSM's guidelines for exercise testing and prescription. 8th ed. Philadelphia (PA): Lippincott Williams & Wilkins; 2009. p. 152–182.
5. Gellish RL, Goslin BR, Olson RE, McDonald A, Russi GD, Moudgil VK. Longitudinal modeling of the relationship between age and maximal heart rate. Med Sci Sport Exerc. 2007 May;39(5):822–9.
6. Rupp. Benefits and risks associated with physical activity. In: American College of Sports Medicine, ed. ACSM's guidelines for exercise testing and prescription. 8th ed. Philadelphia (PA): Lippincott Williams & Wilkins; 2009. p. 1–17

7. American College of Sports Medicine. Position stand: exercise and physical activity for older adults. Med Sci Sports Exerc. 1998 Jun;30(6):992–1008.

8. American College of Sports Medicine. Position stand: the recommended quantity and quality of exercise for developing and maintaining cardiorespiratory and muscular fitness, and flexibility in healthy adults. Med Sci Sports Exerc. 1998 Jun;30(6):975–91.

9. Centers for Disease Control and Prevention (US). Growing stronger: strength training for older adults [Internet]. Atlanta (GA): Department of Health and Human Services (US); [updated 2007 May 22; cited 2008 Feb 4]. 3 p. Available from: http://www.cdc.gov/nccdphp/dnpa/physical/growing_stronger/why.htm

10. Kraemer WJ, Adams K, Cafarelli E, Dudley GA, Dooly C, Feigenbaum MS, Fleck SJ, Franklin B, Fry AC, Hoffman JR, Newton RU, Potteiger J, Stone MH, Ratamess NA, Triplett-McBride T. American College of Sports Medicine position stand on progression models in resistance training for healthy adults. Med Sci Sports Exerc. 2002 Feb;34(2):364–80.

11. Mayo Clinic Staff. Weight training exercises for major muscle groups [Internet]. Rochester (MN): Mayo Foundation for Medical Education and Research. 2008 Jul 4 [cited 2008 Sep 27]. 11 p. Available from: http://www.mayoclinic.com/health/weight-training/SM00041&slide=2

12. NIHSeniorHealth (US). Exercise for older adults: exercises to try—balance exercises [Internet]. Bethesda (MD): National Institute on Aging (US) and US National Library of Medicine. 2002 Mar 19 [reviewed 2005 Jun 29; cited 2008 Feb 8]. 3 p. Available from: http://nihseniorhealth.gov/exercise/balanceexercises/01.html

13. Kibler WB, Press J, Sciascia A. The role of core stability in athletic function. Sports Med. 2006;36(3):189–98.

14. Willardson JM. A periodized approach for core training. ACSM's Health & Fitness J. 2008 Feb;12(1):7–13.

15. Willardson JM. Core stability training: applications to sports conditioning programs. J Strength Cond Res. 2007 Aug;21(3):979–85.

16. Centers for Disease Control and Prevention (US). Physical activity for everyone: measuring physical activity: metabolic equivalent (MET) level [Internet]. Atlanta (GA): Department of Health and Human Services (US); [updated 2007 May 22; cited 2008 Feb 4]. Available from: http://www.cdc.gov/nccdphp/dnpa/physical/measuring/met.htm

17. Ainsworth BE, Haskell WL, Whitt MC, Irwin ML, Swartz AM, Strath SJ, O'Brien WL, Bassett DR, Schmitz KH, Emplaincourt PO, Jacobs DR, Leon AS. Compendium of physical activities: an update of activity codes and MET intensities. Med Sci Sports Exerc. 2000 Sep;32(9suppl):498–516.

CHAPTER 9

Staying Active

Edward M. Phillips, Jennifer Capell, and Steven Jonas

INTRODUCTION

Congratulations! You are now in the "home stretch" of the endurance event that will enable you to effectively provide the exercise prescription for your patients. If you have been able to motivate and assist your patients from the "couch" up to the ACSM/AHA minimum recommended exercise levels, you have achieved the most difficult, yet most important and influential, part of your patient's transformation from a sedentary to an active lifestyle. It is our hope that by this stage both you and your patients are already reaping some of the many mental and physical health benefits of a physically active lifestyle. Your role in your patient's transformation is not quite finished yet, however. You will still need to discuss with him how to *maintain* or even *increase* his new level of fitness. This phase in the exercise prescription is referred to as the "Staying Active" Phase (see Figure 9.1).

Your patients who have reached the ACSM/AHA minimum recommendations (1) should feel proud—they have joined the minority of Americans who are gaining benefits from being physically active. As you have read and will witness when working with some of your patients, this is no small feat; yet, as you know, the benefits cannot be overstated. For many patients, maintaining this minimum level will suffice. However, encouraging them to make periodic increases, or at least changes, in any of the FITT components, will add to the benefits gained from regular exercise.

Some of your patients will have actually "caught the exercise bug" and will be keen to increase their exercise program. For others, you may recommend that for weight loss or other health reasons, their exercise program be increased above the recommended minimum levels. In this chapter, we will first address maintaining an exercise program and will then move to increasing the program. This book is designed to assist you, the clinician, in working with the average patient. If your patient has aspirations of running marathons or competing in other more advanced physical activities, you may want to recommend that he consult racing-specific literature, or even work with a coach or exercise trainer.

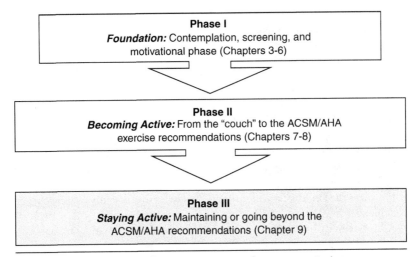

Figure 9.1 • Lifestyle Changes: From Sedentary to Active

As we have said on more than one occasion, in becoming and staying a regular exerciser, one size definitely does not fit all. In Chapter 10, we will provide an alternative approach to providing the exercise prescription—a more structured approach, than the individualized approach that we are taking in this chapter as well as in Chapter 8.

MAINTAINING AN ACTIVE LIFESTYLE

Many of the principles behind maintaining an exercise program are similar to those in beginning a program. A main difference, however, is that once your patient has reached the maintenance stage, she has already incorporated the time to exercise regularly into her daily routine and has begun to reap the benefits of the exercise program. Despite this, your patient will still need to spend some time and effort ensuring that she continues the exercise program. The key to maintaining an exercise program is maintaining motivation. This can be done in a variety of ways, including adding variety to the program, rewarding oneself for reaching certain milestones, taking occasional breaks when necessary, and maintaining the routine and consistency of the program. Please see Chapter 15 for a more extended treatment of "How to Make Regular Exercise Fun."

Motivation and Encouragement

It is not hard to appreciate that your patient may eventually get bored with doing the same exercise routine day after day, month after month. This boredom is not only mental, but also physical. Your patient's muscular and neurological systems also need variety in order to continue to benefit maximally

---

TABLE 9.1 Advantages of Training Using
More Than One Type of Exercise

- Reduces the potential for boredom and lack of motivation through psychological and physical variety
- Promotes overall muscle balance by exercising and developing two or more major muscle groups
- Reduces the risk of injury
- Enables some muscles to recover while others are working
- Increases cardiovascular fitness at a lower risk of overuse or strain to any one major muscle group
- Improves the ability of a wider range of muscles to efficiently use the oxygen in blood
- Adds flexibility to a training program and enables an individual to maintain fitness during the recovery of injuries

---

from exercise. (See Table 9.1, Advantages of Training in More Than One Type of Exercise.) This variety does not have to take the form of an increase in activity, just a change in type. Table 8.3 and Chapter 11 present numerous different types of physical activity that your patients can engage in.

Substituting different activities into an exercise routine, like swimming every Thursday or walking or running outside in the summer and using cardiovascular equipment at the gym in the winter can help your patient to keep up his motivation and to continue to get the maximal physiological benefit from exercising. Alternatively, variety can come from variations in intensity, duration, or routes. For example, your patient could increase his walking speed between certain light poles, could add a hill into one of his routes, or could increase the duration of one or two exercise sessions and decrease a few other sessions, maintaining a frequency of five days each week, for a total of at least 150 minutes each week.

Another strategy that exercisers at all levels can try is the "just getting out the door" approach to dealing with motivationally difficult days. On a day when your patient is feeling "too tired" or "just not motivated" to exercise, ask her to commit to at least starting the workout. This could mean setting an initial goal of walking to the corner of the street or getting to the gym. Often, by the time your patient has taken this initial step, the motivation has kicked in again, and she can persuade herself to keep going a little further. This approach also works during a workout. In this case, after achieving the goal of getting out the door, the patient is encouraged to set a very small goal such as walking to the next lamp post. Then, feeling better having reached the goal, the patient can set another goal of making it to the next lamp post. We have even seen marathon racers use this approach to get through difficult miles in a race—one step, or one tiny goal at a time.

Motivation may also come from pursuing play activities. These may range from competitive sports, to include active video games that involve dancing and simulated sports activities, to trying a new activity or playing actively with the kids. When motivation is lagging, any of these activities may be successful in just getting the patient moving again.

Throughout this process your patient is encouraged to acknowledge his successes and his commitment to a healthier lifestyle. When your patient reaches his goal of exercising at the ACSM/AHA-recommended minimum, you should provide positive reinforcement, and he should find some way to acknowledge himself for his own success. He should also be encouraged to consider setting a new goal, *e.g.,* to maintain the current level for the next six months, to increase his total weekly exercise time from 150 minutes to 200 minutes, or to train for a 5-kilometer race. By setting a new target, even if it is "just" to maintain the same level, he will have something to motivate himself to achieve. Assuming he reaches the new goal, he will have something to celebrate when that next goal is reached.

Keeping Track of Exercise: Logbooks

One way to track progress toward a goal is to regularly record exercise sessions in a logbook. We recommend the use of a simple log from the initiation of an exercise program, as it provides immediate feedback to both the patient and to you. As she progresses into the *staying active* phase, the log becomes more important. It adds motivation and discipline, and can help a patient to get back on track after short breaks in the exercise program.

For patients who decide to progress beyond the ACSM/AHA minimums, it is a useful way to ensure that they do not progress too fast. Running and other sports shops or bookstores offer a variety of logbooks; or your patient can keep track in a diary, or calendar, or electronic PDA. The information tracked depends on the goals of the patient, and can be as simple as number of minutes of exercise on a given day. If the patient so chooses, it can also include other variables, such as the patient's weight and heart rate (resting or exercising heart rate), type of exercise, how the patient felt that day, the intensity of the exercise, or the weather outside.

More sophisticated pedometers and accelerometers can now measure the number of minutes of low-intensity movement, moderate-intensity walking, and vigorous-intensity running and wirelessly record this in a Web site that tracks your patient's activity levels.

Regularity and Consistency

As we have stressed throughout this book, the *regular* part of "regular exercise" is the more difficult component. By reaching the ACSM/AHA minimum exercise recommendations, your patient has likely established a routine in which exercise is part of daily life. Maintaining this consistency in exercising is an important factor in maintaining an active lifestyle. Even the seasoned athlete can fall into the trap of, "Oh well, since I missed my run on the weekend, another day off won't make much difference." Physiologically, missing a few runs will not make a difference in the long run, but psychologically, skipping exercise sessions can lead your patient down the slippery slope toward quitting.

Taking Breaks

At the same time, taking *planned* breaks in one's exercise program are also important. Having stressed the importance of routine and consistency, advocating for breaks may sound like a conflicting message. Planned breaks, such as during a short vacation, or after a goal has been reached, help to revitalize both the mind and the body. The break can act as a reward and as a tool to help re-motivate your patient. A short break (one to two weeks) can be good not only for the mind, but also for the body. When muscles are stressed, particularly through vigorous-intensity exercise, they require recovery time to "assimilate the training"—to recover and strengthen from the activity that they have done. The more intensively your patient is exercising, the more benefit he will get from breaks. This is discussed further in the following section. See Figure 9.2, Step-Wise Exercise Progression that details relative rest periods or breaks every several weeks.

Another time in which rest breaks are necessary is when injury and/or illness occur. Patients should be encouraged to "listen to their bodies," to become more observant of the body's messages telling them when it is getting injured. Patients will need to learn the distinction between Delayed Onset Muscle Soreness (DOMS) (see Chapter 7) that presents as muscle pain beginning approximately 24 hours after a new or increased intensity of activity, and an acute injury that induces pain more quickly. Alternatively, repeatedly stressing a particular joint, such as the dominant elbow in tennis players, can result in overuse injuries. These chronic injuries are due to repetitive stress to the muscles, tendons, bones, and joints. See Table 9.2 Injury Prevention Strategies. Particularly with overuse injuries, the earlier a potential one can be "caught" and rested, the shorter the time that the affected area will have to be rested so that the injury can heal. For example, if a patient starts to notice a "nagging" in her calf when she walks briskly, she should try to find an activity that does not aggravate her calf. This may simply be walking at a slower pace, or may involve trying a different sport, such as swimming, for a week. If these alternatives are not possible or continue to aggravate her calf, she should stop exercising for a short period (one to two weeks), and seek medical attention if the problem does not go away. If she tries to continue exercising through the pain, the injury could worsen, resulting in pain and discomfort during other activities, and a forced break from the aggravating exercise for a longer period (one to two months).

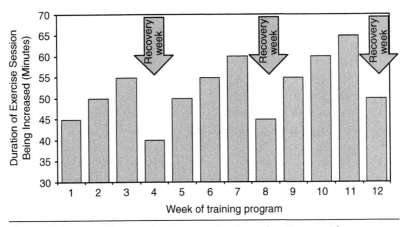

Figure 9.2 • **An Example of Step-wise Exercise Progression**

Clearly, during serious illness, patients should not exercise. During illnesses such as a mild cold or headache, light exercise may be beneficial. As a rule of thumb, if the symptoms of the cold or upper respiratory infection are "above" the shoulders, it is generally fine to continue exercise. However, constitutional symptoms below the neck may best be addressed by rest until they resolve. Elevated resting heart rates (measured upon awakening) are another rough mea-

---

TABLE 9.2 Injury Prevention Strategies

- Increase exercise at a rate of no more that 10% per week.
- Focus on increasing one component of exercise at a time (frequency, or duration, or intensity)
- Include at least two different types of exercise into the weekly routine.
- Include warm-up, cool-down, and stretching components in every work out
- Listen to the body, resting or decreasing intensity, time, or load when discomfort or pain is noted
- Use proper equipment (*e.g.,* supportive footwear, correct bike seat height). Running shoes should be replaced every 350–500 miles.
- Focus on both cardiovascular and resistance training, and include core stability training.
- Follow an exercise program, and keep track of workouts using a logbook.
- Allow room for flexibility in the training program for rest days, recovery workouts, and lighter training weeks.
- Review exercise techniques with an instructor, coach, or exercise professional.

sure that relative rest is indicated. Again, encourage your patient to listen to his body. If exercising makes him feel better during mild illness, there is no reason to stop. If, however, he feels worse exercising, then a break is indicated.

In addition to planned breaks and illness- or injury-related breaks, other obstacles will result in unplanned breaks in your patient's exercise program. Help your patient to accept that these breaks are inevitable and are not damaging to the program unless they result in your patient losing motivation and having difficulty returning to the exercise program, or they lead to de-conditioning which begins after several days of inactivity. Therefore, ensuring that patients are able to get back to their regular exercise routine after a break—either a planned break or an inevitable, unplanned one—should be a priority for both you and your patient.

"Listening" to the Body

You may have heard of athletes being "in tune" with their bodies. This statement can apply to all levels of "athletes"; it just takes awareness and practice. If your patients can learn to listen to the messages their bodies are sending them, they can be effective at minimizing injuries. There are a number of "messages" that the body can send that indicate that an injury or overtraining syndrome is imminent. Mild versions of the symptoms described in Table 9.3, especially nagging discomfort or fatigue, can indicate that the body is in need of rest. Similarly, if exercise becomes stressful (it is usually a stress *reliever* for regular exercisers), it may mean that your patient is letting exercise take control of her life and that a decrease in exercise intensity and/or amount is indicated.

A more objective way in which your patients can "listen" to their bodies is by regularly taking their heart rates. This is commonly done before getting up in the morning (a resting heart rate). Increases in resting heart rate can indicate the onset of illness or overtraining. In such cases, patients should be encouraged to temporarily decrease their exercise level until the heart rate decreases to normal again. A second way your patients can use heart rate to "listen" to their bodies is by wearing a heart rate monitor during exercise (2). Using the monitor, your patient can accurately train within a given heart rate range (see Chapter 8 for general recommendations for exercising heart rate ranges). Regular exercisers should become aware of their resting heart rate upon awakening, their maximal heart rate during vigorous exercise, their heart rate reserve (the difference between these two extremes) and the pattern of heart rate recovery after exercise. If training within a known range is particularly difficult on a given day, it may indicate that the patient is getting sick, or is overtraining.

Injury

Treatment of specific exercise- and sports-related injuries is beyond the scope of this book. We do, however, want to highlight the fact that exercise can increase the chance of developing injuries, particularly intrinsic or overuse injuries. Most of these injuries can be avoided or at least minimized by train-

TABLE 9.3 Physiological and Psychological Signs and Symptoms of Overtraining

Physiological Signs
• Altered resting heart rate and blood pressure
• Chronic fatigue
• Decreased efficiency of movement and physical performance
• Decreased lactate response
• Decreased maximum work capacity
• Frequent nausea/gastrointestinal upsets
• Headaches
• Impaired muscular strength
• Inability to meet previously attained performance standards or criteria
• Increased frequency of respiration
• Insatiable thirst
• Insomnia
• Joint aches and pains
• Lack of appetite
• Lower percent of body fat
• Menstrual disruptions
• Muscle soreness and tenderness
• Prolonged recovery from exercise
• Reappearance of previously corrected mistakes
Psychological Signs
• Changes in personality
• Decreased self-esteem and motivation to work out
• Difficulty concentrating during work, school, or training
• Emotional instability
• Fear of competition
• Feelings of sadness and depression
• General apathy
• "Giving up" when the going gets tough
• Easily distracted during tasks

Adapted from: Kinucan P, Kravitz L. Overtraining: undermining success. ACSM's Health and Fitness J. 2007 Mon; 1(4):8–12; and O'Toole ML. Overreaching and overtraining in endurance athletes. In: Kreider RB, Fry AC, O'Toole ML, editors. Overtraining in Sport, Champaign (IL): Human Kinetics; 1998. 416 p.

ing sensibly and carefully. Table 9.2 highlights some of the important tips for healthy, injury-free training. For a further discussion on exercise-related injuries, please see Chapter 7.

Structural and muscular imbalances can become more problematic as the amount and intensity of exercise increases. Core stability exercises, as described in Chapter 8, can be beneficial for both performance enhancement and injury prevention. These exercises focus on strengthening the postural muscles around the spine, hips, pelvis, abdomen, and proximal portion of the extremities (3). This stability gained in the "core" allows for better alignment and greater mobility in the extremities.

Maintaining a Resistance Training Program

As we discussed in Chapter 7, building up the intensity of a resistance (weight-training) training program can be done by asking your patients to stick to the rule of working against a resistance that is strong (heavy) enough that the patient experiences fatigue after 8–12 repetitions and can complete three sets of these repetitions. With respect to the frequency of the program, we recommend that patients continue with a resistance training program at least twice a week on non-consecutive days. However, research shows that in healthy adults, muscular strength can be maintained by training muscle groups as little as one day each week, provided the training intensity lifted (resistance) is held constant (4). Alternatively, patients may progress to resistance training more than two days per week.

Patients Who Are Still Struggling With Their Exercise Program

Throughout this discussion on maintaining an exercise program, we have assumed that you are working with patients who have at least accepted, if not yet started to positively enjoy, their regular exercise programs. If by the maintenance stage your patient is not at least "tolerating" his exercise program, perhaps you should discuss different types of activity, such as bicycling or golfing instead of walking, or different options in terms of intensity, when, and where to exercise, etc. Please refer back to Chapter 7 or forward to Chapter 11 for a review of these choices.

PROGRESSING BEYOND THE RECOMMENDATIONS

According to the ACSM and the AHA (1):

- "Because of the dose-response relation between physical activity and health, persons who wish to further improve their personal fitness, reduce their risk for chronic diseases and disabilities, or prevent unhealthy weight gain will likely benefit by exceeding the minimum recommended amount of physical activity."
- "Physical activity above the recommended minimum amount provides even greater health benefits."

As we have progressed through the phases of exercise prescription, we have stated that with time, many of your patients will begin to reap the benefits of an active lifestyle. These benefits will inspire some, hopefully many, of your patients to increase their activity level beyond the ACSM/AHA minimum recommendations. Although the primary purpose of this book is to assist clinicians in prescribing regular exercise at a frequency and intensity up to the ACSM/AHA minimum recommendations, we feel that it is important to address some of the issues that may arise when patients want to progress to higher levels of physical activity. This short section is not intended to provide you with a comprehensive understanding of competitive physical activity. If you have patients who have very ambitious exercise goals, they should seek guidance from a professional trainer, coach, exercise physiologist, or sports medicine doctor. As a clinician, however, you should be able to recognize the signs and symptoms of overtraining (see Table 9.3) and to give general advice to patients wanting to increase their exercise level.

The progression of patients beyond the ACSM/AHA minimum exercise levels follows the same principles described in progressing patients to and maintaining patients at this level. These principles include setting goals, maintaining a regular exercise schedule, and finding ways to stay motivated. For more detail on these topics, see Chapter 8 and the earlier sections of Chapter 10.

Rate and Type of Progression

There are some factors that become particularly important as your patient progresses beyond 150 minutes of moderate exercise or 60 minutes of intense exercise per week. Foremost is the rate of progression. The rate at which patients can and will progress depends in part on their medical history and their current health and fitness status. As a general rule, patients should increase their exercise program, in any of its components—frequency, intensity, or time (duration)—at a rate of no more than 10% per week. With the exception of the type of exercise, increases should focus on only one of these components at any given time. For example, if your patient is increasing the duration of her exercise sessions from 30 to 33 minutes, she should avoid simultaneous increases in the frequency or intensity of the exercise.

For many patients, progressing beyond the ACSM/AHA recommendations means increasing intensity. There are many reasons why your patient may want to increase the intensity. One reason may be that exercising at a more vigorous intensity has a greater positive effect on mood. The physiological reason for this is the natural release of mood-enhancing hormones such as endorphins and multiple other neurotransmitters. Also, vigorous-intensity exercise takes less time to reach the same improvement in general health benefits (and caloric expenditure) than lower-intensity exercise. Remember, however, that as we discussed in Chapter 3, not all patients can safely exercise at a vigorous intensity. Such patients can still increase their exercise program above the ACSM/AHA recommendations, but should do so by increasing frequency and duration while maintaining moderate intensity.

Furthermore, patients who were initially assessed to be at moderate risk due to ≥2 cardiac risk factors or high risk due to signs and symptoms of cardiac, pulmonary, or metabolic illness should be reassessed to establish if their active lifestyle (reaching the ACSM/AHA recommended levels) has decreased their risk level. (See Chapter 3.) As a clinician, you have a unique opportunity to offer powerful positive feedback to your patient. If on reassessment your patient's health has improved (*e.g.,* weight loss or lowered blood pressure or cholesterol), providing positive feedback about these changes can be very motivating to your patient.

For a number of reasons (see Table 9.1), combining more than one type of exercise into a weekly training program is beneficial. This is called "cross-training." Two of the primary reasons are that adding variety to an exercise program can help to keep the program interesting and stimulating, and thus, motivating for your patient; and by using different muscles to exercise, your patient can lessen his chance of developing overuse injuries. In Chapter 11, we describe many of the broad range of activities and sports that can be used in an exercise program. In Chapter 12 we present a brief discussion of technique and equipment for some of the more popular sports.

Two approaches to increasing intensity and/or time are racing and joining a club. Patients who enjoy jogging or running, or who are looking for a new challenge, may find road-racing (and triathloning, if they like cycling and swimming, too) to be a fun way to stay motivated and to incorporate a planned rotation of sports into a year-round program. For many activities—from running, to triathlon, to exercise walking—many communities or running stores offer groups to train with. These range from ultracompetitive to "just for fun." Often, a group or club will cater to a range of athletes, from the novice to the expert. Joining such groups can be motivating, inspiring, and a great way to make new friends.

Hydration

Staying hydrated is important for any patient who is engaging in physical activity and becomes more important as your patient increases the intensity and duration of activity. The ACSM recommends that athletes consider hydration in three phases: before, during, and after exercising (5). The goal of prehydration is to begin exercising properly hydrated (neither over- nor underhydrated), with normal plasma electrolyte levels. For many, this will mean drinking fluids, such as water or sports drinks, a few hours prior to exercising to enable adequate fluid absorption. Once exercise begins, patients should try to drink small amounts regularly, especially if exercising over one hour. After exercise, patients should drink enough to replace lost water and electrolytes. In order to maintain an adequate fluid balance, your patient will usually need to drink before he becomes thirsty.

Individuals lose water and electrolytes at different rates depending on their physiological makeup, environment, and clothing. Therefore, the ACSM does not give precise recommendations as to how much liquid patients should be drinking. It recommends drinking to prevent excessive loss, and to replace fluid and electrolyte loss. To determine how much fluid is lost during exercise, patients can weigh themselves before and after a workout. If the patient is lighter at the end of the exercise session, the weight lost is most likely due to fluid loss and, therefore, the amount lost is the amount that should be replaced. Similarly, if the patient weighs more after exercising, he has likely consumed too much liquid. Consumption of too much liquid, particularly water, can result in hyponatremia, a rare but potentially dangerous condition. A second method that patients can use to monitor their fluid intake is to check their urine output and color. A well-hydrated patient should produce a large amount of light-colored (neither clear nor dark yellow) urine.

When exercising for shorter durations (less that one hour) or at moderate intensities, drinking water will usually suffice. However, as patients increase the intensity and duration of exercise, consuming liquids that contain both carbohydrates and electrolytes can enhance both performance and recovery.

Following a Planned Training Program

The following are a set of general concepts that you and your patients can use in planning their training programs. (We get into more specifics for the leisure-time scheduled approach in Chapter 10.) Throughout this book, we have stressed the importance of helping your patients establish a regular schedule for exercising. As your patient begins to increase his exercise program, this point remains important. Due to time restrictions, some patients will be tempted to condense all of their training into one or two sessions. Again, spreading exercise sessions over at least three days is recommended.

Similar to patients just beginning or maintaining an exercise program, keeping to a planned exercise schedule helps to keep patients motivated, and helps them to reach their goals. For patients moving beyond the minimum recommendations, a planned schedule is also important to prevent injuries and to assist them in focusing on the desired components at the desired time.

As we discussed, your patient's training program should focus on increasing one component at a time (frequency, intensity or duration). There are different approaches to increasing each component. For example, if your patient begins at the ACSM/AHA recommendations for vigorous activity (three 20-minute sessions each week), she may keep two of the sessions at 20 minutes duration, while increasing the third by 10% a week. Before the difference between the two shorter and one longer session becomes too great, she may increase each of the shorter two, while maintaining the length of the longer one. Your patient will need to find a balance between making changes to the program and maintaining a degree of consistency. Having a pre-planned training program will help your patient to keep track of the changes.

Similarly, throughout the year or the training season, your patient will want to focus on different aspects of training—speed, strength, flexibility, endurance, etc. A training schedule will help your patient to plan these changes. Focusing on different components at different times, as well as scheduling in harder and easier weeks, is known as "phase training" or "periodization." These changes help to minimize overuse injuries, as well as to maximize the effects of training.

Throughout the program, both rest days and active recovery days should be scheduled in. Active recovery days are those in which your patient will be active, but will exercise at a lower intensity and possibly for a shorter duration than usual. These lighter workouts help the body to recover physiologically and psychologically. Specifically, active recovery days help to decrease lactic acid in muscles and to promote relaxation (6, 7). Active recovery is particularly important after high-intensity workouts, including races. Although there are different ways of structuring an exercise program, a common one is a step-wise increase: patients gradually increase their program over a period of three weeks, and then follow this with a lighter recovery week. This four-week plan is then repeated from a starting point that is higher than the start of the first repetition, but not as high as the final (third) week of the cycle. Figure 9.2 illustrates this sequence.

Periodically, patients will need to miss a training session or will want to change either the time or the date of a particular session due to travel, weather, or other commitments. Allowing for some flexibility within the training program is advisable. Whether or not to make up missed training sessions will depend on your patient's preferences and time. If the training session missed is a key session, such as the session in which the patient is increasing his training, making up the session is more important than "regular" sessions. If several sessions are missed, instead of making them all up, the training program may need to be revised. This is inevitable from time to time, and should be seen as an expected event.

Warm-Up and Cool-Down

Virtually all exercise authorities, including the ACSM (1), recommend at least a 5–10-minute warm-up period at the beginning of each exercise session and a 3–5-minute cool-down at the end. The more intense the exercise session, the more important the warm-up and cool-down phases of an exercise session are. Consider at the extreme, a 100-meter sprinter jumping on the track for a race without warming up or cooling down. To perform optimally, and injury-free, muscles need to be "eased" in and out of an intense session.

The warm-up and cool-down phases usually, but not always, consist of the same exercise, *e.g.,* running, done at a lower intensity, by starting with a brisk walk or slow jog. By stopping suddenly, without a cool-down period, the heart continues to pump hard, but the leg muscles are no longer contracting to help force the blood back to the heart. This can cause blood pooling in the lower extremities, leaving the internal organs and brain temporarily short of adequate blood supply. The cool-down period also helps prevent the buildup of lactic acid in muscles. Lactic acid is a chemical by-product of exercise that may increase muscle soreness.

As we discussed in Chapter 7, stretching is also recommended after the warm-up or the cool-down phase, but not prior to the warm-up, when the muscles are still cold. Research surrounding the type and duration of stretching is still inconclusive; however, it is still widely recommended to improve range of motion and physical function (8). Although it is unclear whether stretching has acute benefits on physical activity, it is likely that stretching will help to counter the loss in range of motion associated with aging (8).

Measuring Time Versus Distance

Depending on where your patient obtains her training program from, the duration or time for each session may be given in distance or time (*e.g.,* "run 4 miles" instead of "run 35 minutes"). Either method is appropriate; however, we advocate prescribing exercise in minutes, not miles. Measuring in time may be easier for your patients, as this simply requires a watch, rather than a GPS or pedometer. For some patients, thinking in terms of miles will be intimidating; while for others, knowing the distance that they are covering will be motivating. Nevertheless, the message to those starting out—"it's the minutes, not the miles"—can apply to the more active patients as well. When measuring distance, however, your patient may have a tendency to think in terms of speed (*e.g.,* minutes per mile, or miles per hour) which may tempt her to increase her intensity more quickly than she has planned. Thus, it is sometimes useful for patients to have at least a rough idea of how fast they are training. In order to determine this, your patient can go to an outdoor track and time how long it takes to complete four laps in the inside lane. This will give her the time to complete one mile. Unless she is training to exercise competitively, speed should not be the primary focus of his training.

For some of your patients, however, achieving a certain distance by signing up for a race or, at first, a "fun run" may prove to be motivating. The prospect of a measurable goal of having to run a specific distance by a given date, or of losing the entrance fee, or of experiencing the "defeat" of not being able to participate in the event can be excellent sources of motivation. Participating in a race does not have to mean competing in the race. On virtually every weekend in warmer months different groups hold runs for charity. These are usually friendly and not very competitive. Alternatively, bigger races that are competitive for the frontrunners are generally friendly for the rest of the field.

Overtraining

For most of this book, we have focused on a "more is better" approach to exercise, encouraging your patient to walk two blocks if he is currently only walking one, or pushing your patient to exercise moderately five days each week instead of three or four. You will, however, possibly encounter patients who have the potential to exercise too much. The risk of *overtraining* is of relevance only to elite athletes. This is distinguished from *overuse* injuries described in the Injury section above. There is no set threshold beyond which patients are exercising too much, and you will likely encounter athletes who are training at a significantly higher level than we discuss here. We leave the management of highly trained athletes to coaches, sports medicine specialists, and to sport-specific books that deal with performance.

Similar to medicines, there are two "maximum doses," both of which vary with a patient's physiology and fitness level. The first maximum can be described as a *ceiling* effect. This is a point at which further activity will result in minimal additional benefit to the patient's general health. For the average healthy adult patient, this threshold will occur at approximately 3,500 to 4,000 kilocalories of energy expenditure per week in exercise. This would translate to walking or running approximately 30 to 40 miles per week or to vigorous-intensity exercise for at least seven to eight hours per week. The second maximum is a point at which your patient begins to cause more damage than benefit by exercising. This is known as *overtraining* and is characterized by a variety of signs and symptoms, as presented in Table 9.3.

It can be difficult for patients who are overtraining to recognize and accept that they are doing so. It is your role to help patients to identify signs and symptoms that result from overtraining and to highlight the negative effects that overtraining can have on both physical performance and on health. The likelihood of overtraining can be minimized through the following ways:

- Set realistic goals and know your limits
- Increase exercise intensity, duration, or frequency at a rate of ≤10% or less per week
- Listen to the body
- Follow a training plan that includes rest days
- Keep track of exercise sessions (use an exercise log)

Some of these points have already been discussed (rate of progression, following a training plan, and keeping track of exercise sessions). In the following section, we will cover the remaining points.

Set Realistic Goals and Know Your Limits

By now, your patient has reached his first goal of achieving the ACSM/AHA-recommended exercise minimums and is actively moving on to further goals of increased exercise. From here, it is equally important to set realistic and achievable goals. Such goals are important to maintain motivation, to have something to work towards, and to reward oneself once the goal is reached. However, when setting goals, your patient needs to be realistic about what is attainable and how to avoid an injury. Huge improvements in speed, strength, muscular bulk, flexibility, skill, and gracefulness can be achieved through training and practice, but this practice takes time and dedication. Conversely, few of your patients have the genetic makeup or the dedication to enable them to become a world-class athlete, no matter how much training they do. Depending on each patient's personality, you will need to find a balance between motivating and encouraging patients to push themselves beyond their perceived limits, and to help other patients set less ambitious and more achievable goals.

CONCLUSION

As with most things in life, balance and moderation are keys to exercise. Either too much or too little can be harmful. Helping your patients find a balance that is right for them, whether it is at the ACSM/AHA-recommended minimum or at running marathons, is an important and valuable skill for you as a clinician. Similar to other types of medicine, if your patients' exercise prescription becomes complicated as a result of confounding medical conditions or because of high exercise aspirations, we recommend that you refer your patient on to other medical or exercise professionals.

In this chapter, we have discussed how to assist your patient to maintain or to increase an exercise program. Although it is inevitable that your patient will encounter challenges that may disrupt his training program, it is important that your patient tries to follow a regular training schedule. As the amount (frequency, duration, or intensity) increases, so does the chance of overuse injuries. Help your patient to learn to listen to his body and to be aware of the early warning signs of injury. Finally, as with any area of medicine, if your patient's situation becomes more complicated than with which you are comfortable, refer him to a medical or exercise professional.

Throughout this book, we have tried to give you choices as to how best to prescribe exercise to your patient. In the next chapter, we will give you another choice. In contrast to Chapters 8 and 9, which give general principles and parameters for exercise prescription, Chapter 10 will walk you through a specific leisure-time scheduled exercise program, beginning with a sedentary patient and progressing somewhat beyond the ACSM/AHA-recommended minimum exercise levels. In the following chapters, you will also learn how to assist patients in choosing the sport/activity that's right for them (Chapter 11), in learning about technique and equipment (Chapter 12), and in how to have fun while exercising regularly, to maintain their interest and motivation (Chapter 15).

References

1. Haskell WH, Lee IM, Pate RR, Powell KE, Blair SN, Franklin BA, Macera CA. Physical activity and public health: updated recommendations for adults from the American College of Sports Medicine and the American Heart Association. Circulation. 2007 Aug;116(9):1081–93.

2. Edwards S. Heart rate monitoring guidebook. Sacramento (CA): Heart Rate®; 2005. 257 p.

3. Kibler WB, Press J, Sciascia A. The role of core stability in athletic function. Sports Med. 2006;36(3):189–198.

4. Kraemer WJ, Adams K, Cafarelli E, Dudley GA, Dooly C, Feigenbaum MS, Fleck SJ. American College of Sports Medicine position stand: progression models in resistance training for healthy adults. Med Sci Sports Exerc. 2002 Feb;34(2):364–80.

5. American College of Sports Medicine; Sawka MN, Burke LM, Eichner ER, Maughan RJ, Montain SJ, Stachenfeld NS. American College of Sports Medicine position stand: exercise and fluid replacement. Med Sci Sports Exerc. 2007 Feb;39(2):377–90.

6. Micklewright D, Beneke R, Gladwell V, Sellens MH. Blood lactate removal using combined massage and active recovery. Med Sci Sports Exerc. 2003 May; 35(Suppl 1):S317.

7. Suzuki M, Umeda T, Nakaji S, Shimoyama T, Mashiko T, Sugawara K. Effect of incorporating low intensity exercise into the recovery period after a rugby match. Br J Sports Med. 2004 Aug:38(4)1;436–40.

8. Garber ME. Exercise prescription. In: American College of Sports Medicine, ed. ACSM's guidelines for exercise testing and prescription. 8th edition. Philadelphia (PA): Lippincott Williams & Wilkins; 2009. p. 152–182.

CHAPTER 10

TSTEP: Training Programs by the Minute

Steven Jonas

INTRODUCTION

In the previous three chapters, we outlined the general principles of exercise prescription, enabling you to design a personalized exercise program for your patient. In this chapter, we use many of those principles to provide you with a specific program that your patients may want to follow in order to either begin exercising and then progress to the ACSM/AHA/HHS-recommended levels, or to advance beyond the minimum recommendations. As with many aspects of this book, we are leaving the choice up to you. It may well be the case that some of your patients will respond better to a specific program such as the ones presented in this chapter, while others will benefit more from a personalized program designed based on the principles and parameters discussed in Chapters 8 and 9. We can use the same flow diagram presented in Figure 10.1 to illustrate your patients' potential progression as they transform their lifestyle from sedentary to active.

Whether you are using the principles-and-parameters approach to exercise prescription (Chapters 8 and 9) or the specific-prescription approach presented in this chapter, it is important that you review the basic concepts of exercise prescription, as presented in Chapter 7. If you are working with a patient who is at the stage of maintaining or exceeding the ACSM/AHA/HHS recommendations it will also be important to review the general information in Chapter 9, covering topics such as hydration and overtraining, even if you are using the approach presented in this chapter.

The specific training program that we will focus on in this chapter is called The Scheduled Training Exercise Program, or TSTEP. It was designed by Dr. Steven Jonas and has been in use for some years now (1–4). The training precepts on which it is based were established some time ago by the world-renowned middle-distance running coach from the University of Oregon, Bill Bowerman (5). Adapted from Coach Bowerman's famous "Ten Principles," Table 10.1 highlights the seven key principles for TSTEP.

In this approach you and your patient can pick and choose among the various training schedules provided, depending on the patient's current fitness

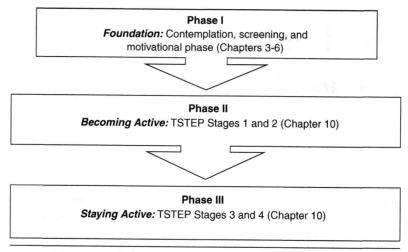

Figure 10.1 • Lifestyle Changes: From Sedentary to Active Using a Specific Training Program

level, her goals, and other considerations. Please note that while the advice and counsel offered in this chapter is aimed primarily at patients who are engaged in leisure-time scheduled exercise, there is plenty of information that will be helpful for those patients following the lifestyle exercise route as well.

TSTEP is designed for use by leisure-time scheduled regular exercisers at any level (up to race training), from at-scratch beginner to experienced sportsperson, who are choosing this mode of regular exercise. For the beginner, it provides an easy, gradual entry into the world of regular exercise that, in terms of graduated time and effort, is as painless as possible (see Table 10.2). The Program in Table 10.3 is designed to get your patient to the ACSM/AHA/HHS

TABLE 10.1 The Seven Key Principles for TSTEP

1. Training must be regular, according to a long-term program.
2. The watchword is moderation.
3. The workload must be balanced, and overtraining must be avoided.
4. Goals should be clearly established, they must be understood, and they must be realistic.
5. Training schedules should be set up with a hard/easy rotation, both from day to day and, more generally, over time.
6. Regular rest should be scheduled.
7. Whenever possible, working out should be fun

TABLE 10.2 The Scheduled Training Exercise Program—
Stage I: Introductory Program

Week	M	T	W	Th	F	S	S	Total	Comments

	(Times in Minutes)								
	Day								
Week	**M**	**T**	**W**	**Th**	**F**	**S**	**S**	**Total**	**Comments**
1	Off	10	Off	10	Off	Off	10	30	Ordinary
2	Off	10	Off	10	Off	Off	10	30	walking
3	Off	20	Off	20	Off	Off	20	60	Ordinary
4	Off	20	Off	20	Off	Off	20	60	walking
5	Off	20	Off	20	Off	Off	20	60	Fast
6	Off	20	Off	20	Off	Off	20	60	walking
7	Off	20	Off	20	Off	Off	30	70	Fast
8	Off	20	Off	20	Off	Off	30	70	walking
9	Off	20	Off	20	Off	Off	20	60	PaceWalking™
10	Off	20	Off	20	Off	Off	30	70	
11	Off	20	Off	30	Off	Off	30	80	PaceWalking™
12	Off	20	Off	30	Off	Off	30	80	
13	Off	30	Off	30	Off	Off	30	90	PaceWalking™

weekly-minimum recommendation for regular exercise of moderate intensity. For the experienced regular exerciser, it provides a comfortable, easy-to-maintain program that will keep him in shape without overdoing it (see Table 10.4).

The overall Program is rigorous in its requirements for consistency and regularity. Nevertheless, it maintains a degree of internal flexibility. Within it, one can move around from high-volume weeks to lower volume ones, depending on other needs and fitness level. However, before getting to those details, let's go over once again getting started on the road to becoming and being a regular exerciser, since how your patient goes about that is critical to success. Along with very careful, self-developed goal-setting, getting started right is an absolutely critical part of the whole enterprise. As we have said before and will say again, *the hard part of regular exercise is the regular, not the exercise.* Therefore, the focus in getting active should be *first* on the *regular,* not the *exercise.* Whether one is using the leisure-time scheduled or the lifestyle exercise approach, your first concentration should be to help your patient find the time and make the time that will be set aside for exercise in their life on a regular basis.

For those using the lifestyle exercise approach, that could be determining to climb the stairs part or all the way to the office, at first twice a week, but on

TABLE 10.3 The Scheduled Training Exercise Program—Stage II: Developmental Program. To reach the ACSM/AHA/HHS Minimum for Moderate Physical Activity: 30 Minutes, 5 Times/Week

	(Times in Minutes)							
	Day							
Week	M	T	W	Th	F	S	S	Total
1	Off	Off	Off	Off	Off	Off	Off	Off
2	Off	20	Off	20	Off	Off	20	60
3	Off	20	Off	20	Off	10	20	70
4	Off	20	Off	20	Off	20	20	80
5	Off	20	Off	20	Off	20	30	90
6	Off	20	Off	30	Off	20	30	100
7	Off	30	Off	30	Off	20	30	110
8	Off	30	Off	30	Off	30	30	120
9	Off	30	Off	30	Off	30	30	120
10	Off	30	Off	20	Off	30	20	120
11	Off	30	30	30	Off	30	30	150
12	Off	30	30	30	Off	30	30	150
13	Off	30	30	30	Off	30	30	150

given days; similarly, parking at the far end of the parking lot, at first twice a week, on given days. The idea is to first get used to the pattern. Then, one can start expanding it. Similarly, with leisure-time scheduled exercise, for most people starting from scratch, the first step should be just getting out there and walking, up and down or around the block, for ten minutes or so, three times a week, for a couple of weeks. That's just plain walking at their regular pace. Not fast, no sweat, no hard breathing. The critical element is to do it on a schedule, like Monday-Wednesday-Friday, or Tuesday-Thursday-Saturday, or Wednesday-Saturday-Sunday, at a given time each time.

As we have noted time and again, with these first steps, the focus should be not on the exercise, but on the *habit of exercising:* setting aside the needed time, whether that is first thing in the morning, or just after the kids are off to school, or on lunch break, or right after work, or before or (a bit) after dinner. Then, once the habit has been established, one gradually expands the amount of time spent and usually picks a single sport or activity to focus on, at least at

TABLE 10.4 The Scheduled Exerciser Training Program—Stage III: Going to the Next Level. Longer Workouts, 4 Times per Week, Reaching 3 Hours

	(Times in Minutes)							
	Day							
Week	M	T	W	Th	F	S	S	Total
1	Off	Off	Off	Off	Off	Off	Off	Off
2	Off	30	Off	40	Off	30	50	150
3	Off	30	Off	40	Off	40	50	160
4	Off	40	Off	40	Off	40	50	170
5	Off	30	Off	50	Off	40	60	180
6	Off	30	Off	40	Off	30	50	150
7	Off	40	Off	30	Off	30	60	160
8	Off	40	Off	40	Off	40	50	170
9	Off	30	Off	50	Off	40	60	180
10	Off	30	Off	40	Off	30	50	150
11	Off	40	Off	30	Off	30	60	160
12	Off	40	Off	40	Off	40	50	170
13	Off	30	Off	50	Off	40	60	180

the beginning. These programs then detail recommended increases in intensity and frequency. Now to those detailed programs.

TSTEP: AN OVERVIEW

The Overall Framework for TSTEP

TSTEP has four Stages, each 13 weeks long. For each Stage, a specific Exercise Program is presented, each providing a suggested schedule of minutes per day and days per week for the 13 weeks of the Program. You will find the tables for these Programs on pp. 153, 154, 155, and 156.

The first Stage introduces your patient to regular exercise (Table 10.2). Its Program requires just three workouts per week. The second develops your patient's abilities and skills as a regular exerciser (Table 10.3). Its Program enables your patient to begin building up strength and endurance, the primary physical requirements for success in this endeavor. It enables your patient to

TABLE 10.5 The Scheduled Exerciser's Training Program—Program IV: Really Getting into It and Getting Ready to Race. Establishing 4 Hours per Week, Over 5 Workouts

| Week | (Times in Minutes) Day | | | | | | | Total |
	M	T	W	Th	F	S	S	
1	Off	Off	Off	Off	Off	Off	Off	Off
2	Off	30	40	Off	30	40	40	180
3	Off	30	30	Off	30	40	50	190
4	Off	30	40	Off	40	40	50	200
5	Off	30	40	Off	30	50	60	210
6	Off	40	30	Off	30	50	70	220
7	Off	30	50	Off	30	60	60	230
8	Off	30	50	Off	30	60	70	240
9	Off	30	40	Off	30	50	60	210
10	Off	40	30	Off	30	50	70	220
11	Off	30	50	Off	30	60	60	230
12	Off	30	50	Off	30	60	70	240
13	Off	30	50	Off	30	70	60	240

reach the ACSM minimum recommendation of 30 minutes of moderate-intensity exercise, five times per week. These first two Stages correspond with the second Phase of lifestyle change that we have been describing throughout this book: the Becoming Active Phase (see Figure 10.1). The third Stage offers your patient the opportunity to go to the next level, dropping down in weekly frequency by one, but increasing in total time, getting up to three hours per week (Table 10.4). The final offering here (Table 10.5) takes your patient up to 4 hours per week and back up to five workouts. Now she is "really getting into it" and possibly "getting ready to race" (see Chapter 12). The choice is hers. Just remember. These Programs are designed to help your patient become a regular exerciser by *changing herself gradually, taking small, easy, steps, one step at a time.*

What Are the Sports or Activities Might be Used, and How Might They be Grouped?

The sports and activities are discussed in detail in the next chapter. Here we just have some general comments.

The variety of physical activities and sports that regular exercisers engage in can be conveniently divided into two types, termed "forward motion," and "in place." The forward motion sports include, for example, PaceWalking™ (our term for "exercise walking," "power walking," "fitness walking"; see Chapters 11 and 12), running, cycling, rowing, and swimming, all of which, given the right equipment and venues, can be done either indoors (on machines) or outdoors. The in-place activities and sports include aerobic dance, stepping, weight-training, stair-climbing, and using some version of the elliptical trainer. These are usually done indoors.

Because ordinary walking is the best way to start if your patient has never previously been a regular exerciser (as has been pointed out in this book on more than one occasion) TSTEP's Stage I begins with it, and then moves on to fast walking, before getting to PaceWalking™. Ordinary walking is good for openers, whether your patient intends to go on to a one sport/activity program or are thinking about one which will include two or more sports at the same time (see the section on PaceTraining at the end of this chapter). It is also best to start with walking if your patient hasn't yet made up his mind about what he is going to be doing later on.

At the same time, your patient should not think that she is being put into some walking straight-jacket. If she would like to start off her TSTEP by doing easy aerobic dancing at home in front of the TV for ten minutes at a time or by going to the gym to do her minutes, slowly, on a stairclimber or elliptical trainer, or doing some gentle jogging outside—that's fine too. These Programs are provided for your patients as guides. If they want to and feel that they can safely move through at a faster pace than presented in the tables, then let them do it. A very important element of this whole approach is that your patient should know: *You* [the patient] *are in control of what you actually do.*

Time and Distance

Whether your patient is doing a forward-motion or an in-place sport or activity, TSTEP workouts are measured in minutes. To get the primary benefits of regular exercise, all your patient needs to do is put in the time. Distance is immaterial. Whether their exercise is non-aerobic or aerobic, the more time spent, the more benefit they will get in terms of improving their fitness level, burning calories, raising their resting metabolic rate, managing stress, improving musculoskeletal strength and flexibility and clarity of thought. With the forward-motion sports, if your patients measure their workouts by time, they don't need to be concerned with how far they have gone, only for how long they have gone. They need only a stopwatch/chronometer, not a wrist-mounted global positioning system (GPS—and yes, there are such things).

Thinking in miles instead of minutes leads to thinking about absolute speed. The latter can be a negative factor for the regular exerciser. Thinking about absolute speed can lead to frustration when one's maximum is reached speed in PaceWalking™, let's say, and, like many of us, one finds that one is just not very fast compared to others'. Thinking about speed can also lead to injury if one tries to go fast when one is not physically capable of doing so. For the regular exerciser, the only important speed is the one that one is comfortable with.

If your patient has decided to exercise aerobically (see below, pp. 158–162), the only speed she needs to be concerned with is the one she needs to reach so that her heart rate is in the moderate-intensity range (see Table 7.1). How that speed compares with anyone else's or to some absolute standard is unimportant. If someone asks her how far she goes in her workouts, she just answers in minutes, not miles. There are also practical advantages to measuring workouts in minutes, rather than in miles. If she exercises outdoors, she doesn't have to measure or lay out specific courses. She will probably find one or two routes that she likes so much that she will want to do them over and over again, for pleasure, not necessity. But she doesn't have to have any definite routes. Using the minutes method, for a 30-minute outdoor workout she can simply PaceWalk™ or jog or cycle away from the house for 15 minutes and then just retrace that route at about the same pace.

GETTING INTO TSTEP

Introduction

As noted previously on more than one occasion, it's the *regular,* not the *exercise,* that is the hard part for most people who are not presently regular exercisers, and even for some who already are. That is, it is not the activity itself that's tough, but doing it on a regular basis—making, finding, and keeping available the time in one's busy life and schedule to exercise. Once the pattern is established, and that may take some time, then your patient simply has to design or adopt/adapt a program which will help him to achieve his goal, while developing and maintaining enjoyment, dealing with potential boredom, and not getting injured.

What Is the Roadmap for the Program?

The four Stages mentioned connect with each other in a logical manner. If your patient has never exercised regularly before, or hasn't done it in a long time, he should definitely start off with Stage I (see also Chapter 8). The tables show how many minutes should be done for each workout. Within the requirements for consistency and regularity, however, the Programs do not have to be followed rigidly. They are guides, not specific instructions. Changes can be made to suit different needs and life-schedules, as long as one generally stays within TSTEP Principles.

If a session is missed, and your patient would like to make up the time (which they certainly do not have to do for the occasional miss), it should not be all added onto just one other workout session. The make-up minutes should be spread out over several of them. Or your patient can put in an extra session. It will not hurt to do two workouts in a row during the week. If bad weather or travel or an early morning meeting causes Tuesday to be missed, that work-out can be on Wednesday and the Thursday workout can still be done as well. Also, it won't hurt to do your workouts at different times on different days.

Furthermore, while the Program is designed to provide a slow, easy intro-duction to regular exercise, after giving the idea some careful thought, it can cer-tainly be moved through at a quicker pace than the one provided for. If one already has some exercise experience, Stage I can be skipped entirely. Or your patient may start Stage I and find himself progressing more rapidly than the schedule calls for. In this case, he should not feel constrained to follow the sched-ule minute-by-minute, day-by-day, and week-by-week. Minutes and workouts can be added; the early weeks of ordinary walking can be skipped; your patient can go right on to Stage II. Some people become very enthusiastic very early on and move ahead very quickly. They should just be careful not to overdo it.

Stage I: The Introductory Program

The Introductory Program, (see Table 10.2) begins at 30 minutes for the week and finishes up at an hour and a half, in total. If your patient has never done any exercise, or hasn't done it for a long time, it's a good idea to begin here. This Program is designed to gradually ease her into a regular schedule of workouts, to help her limber up slowly, minimizing the risk of pain or injury. As noted, because PaceWalking™ (see Chapter 11 for a discussion of the tech-nique) is ideal as the basic long-term sport for TSTEP, this Stage concludes with a focus on PaceWalking™. But, of course, the Program will work with any sport or other physical activity you choose.

For the first two weeks, your patient will just be going out for a 10-minute walk, three times each week. He should not be concerned with heart rate or speed. Just walk comfortably for ten minutes. (Doing a bit more if he feels like it certainly won't hurt, but he doesn't have to.) At this point he has nothing else to do but to become regular. He needs to get that exercise schedule into his calendar and stick with it. He can arise a bit earlier in the morning if nec-essary, get out of bed when he might not be quite ready to do so, put on his exercise outfit (see Chapter 11 also for advice on shoes and clothing), and go out—just to walk, and do it even if the weather isn't quite right.

Right now, right up front, she has a chance to get in control and stay in control. She has had that first crack at healthy immediate gratification. No, on this Program she won't lose 20 pounds in two weeks, or be ready to run a marathon in two months, or challenge for the Ms. Universe title in two years. It's not that kind of gratification we're talking about. *It's the gratification of the mind.* In two weeks she can begin to take control of her life, add something new, and take the first big step toward making regular exercise a part of it. In two weeks she can show herself that she is ready to take responsibility for how she looks, how she feels, and how she feels about herself. That can give her gratification aplenty. For the next two weeks, she will go out for 20 minutes at a time, still just walking, at a pace that is comfortable for her. She will continue her loosening-up process, continue getting used to being on a schedule of workouts. But her primary focus will remain on establishing the regularity of exercising in her life.

In weeks five through eight, your patient continues with ordinary walking, but will try going a bit faster. We are still not talking about PaceWalking™ here. He shouldn't be concerned with armswing or foot placement. He should, however, try to begin working on developing a steady, smooth, easy rhythm for walking. Getting into a rhythm makes walking fun, easy, and gets your patient ready to take up PaceWalking™.

In week nine of Stage I, your patient starts PaceWalking™ (again, see the Chapter 11 for the description of the technique). He should not be concerned with all the technical points at this time. He should just hone in on the following four: keeping the upper body relaxed, avoiding scrunched shoulders; gradually developing a strong armswing; with each step coming down firmly on the heel, rolling forward to a nice, lifting push-off from the toes; and developing a smooth, steady rhythm. After a bit of practice, your patient will start to become comfortable with the gait. Obviously, he won't worry about speed. Just remember, at this time he is still focusing primarily on incorporating regular exercise into his lifestyle.

Stage II: The Developmental Program

Beginning in week three of the Developmental Program (Table 10.3), there are four workouts per week, two each on weekdays and weekend days. In terms of time required, this Program is obviously more demanding than Program I. However, please note that in each week, one-half or more of the total minutes are scheduled on the two weekend days. This makes life easier for the regular exerciser who is working outside the home. (By the way, if your patient's schedule requires that he works on the weekends, these Programs can certainly be rearranged to meet such needs.)

In this Program, your patient will develop her regular exercising to the point where at the end of it she is doing the ACSM/AHA/HHS-recommended minimum of 2.5 hours of moderate-intensity exercise per week, over five workout sessions. By the Program's end, she will have been on an exercise schedule for up to 26 weeks. For most people that means exercise has become a regular part of their life and they should be able to continue doing it indefinitely. Notice that, following TSTEP Principle number six, this Program begins with a week off. (For regular exercisers off-time is scheduled on a regular basis, as we have noted more than once.) By so doing, you are helping to prevent exercise burnout. The break gives the mind and body some rest. Don't worry, they won't lose their conditioning with a week or two off. Your patient is developing; a new physical shape. It will certainly not revert to its pre-TSTEP contours in that amount of time.

Going through the Program in some detail, after the week off, there is a light week, in total time well below the last one of Stage I. After that, the weekly time requirement builds steadily throughout this Program. But even so, the workout lengths vary within each week, following the Bowerman hard-easy principle. The Stage II Program weekly workout time peaks at three hours. Most people can comfortably and safely get to that level. Whatever your patient's intermediate objective, in the latter part of this Stage he may well be working on getting his technique down and his speed up. He certainly will be getting into better shape than he has ever been in. If he is exercising at a moderate intensity, he will probably find that he will have to work harder in order to boost his heart rate above the minimum for vigorous aerobic activity. If he is PaceWalking™, he will see how important armswing really is.

When she finishes Stage II of the Program, she should congratulate herself. She will have become a regular exerciser. She may well have learned a new sport. She is becoming healthier, and, if she has chosen to do so, aerobically fit as well. Her stamina and endurance will have increased significantly. She may even have discovered that she has some previously undiscovered talent in the sport(s) she has chosen. Such a discovery could open up whole new vistas for her. Perhaps most importantly, she continues to feel better and feel better about herself.

Perhaps it's time for her to reward herself for all of her discipline and hard work. Perhaps she will go out and buy that great sports outfit she has been eyeing. Perhaps she will get away for a special weekend in the country, with or without exercise as a part of it. Or, dare we say it, perhaps she will consume that double hot-fudge sundae that she has been dutifully putting off having for the last three months!

Stages III and IV: Going to the Next Level

Your patient has made it! Six months ago (and for certain folks fewer than that) he was able to mobilize his motivation and decide that he was indeed going to make regular exercise a part of his life. He took control. He took responsibility for his shape. He stopped making excuses, he stopped putting it off until tomorrow, and he got over his fear of failure. He went out and did it. Now he is ready for Stage III of TSTEP if he wants to go there.

In this Stage, she will ramp it up to three hours per week, in four workouts (see Table 10.4). If she feels like going beyond that at some point, she is "Really Getting into It" and possibly even starting to think about racing in one of the distance-sports (see Table 10.5). She, of course, has the option of mixing and matching among Stages II–IV throughout the year.

Once again this Program begins with a week off, to feel good about oneself, resting and relaxing a bit. Your patient will average about 2.75 hours per week over the remaining 12 weeks of this Program. At a moderate level of intensity, that is just slightly over the minimum time recommended by the American College of Sports medicine. Very few regular exercisers who get into a sport actually do only the minimum. Most people who get into sports, aerobic or not, seem naturally drawn to do more. Nevertheless, he may well find 2.5 to 3 hours per week to be a comfortable, productive amount.

Following the obligatory first week OFF, "Really Getting into It" (Table 10.4) provides for an average of about 3.5 hours per week spread over 5 workouts per week for the 12 weeks. (With this schedule one could, for example, do a Sprint triathlon at a modest rate of speed.) For the busy person, although this Program provides for more minutes per week, more than half the total minutes in it are concentrated in the two weekend days.

If she is doing her workouts at least at a moderate aerobic intensity, using this Program she will be over the "Three Hour Max" for health benefits. Thus, many regular exercisers will find this Program to be very comfortable on a permanent basis. She certainly could modify this to do the time in just four workouts if she wants to, should she find that after reaching this level an average of about one hour per session is a comfortable workout time for her. If she prefers to maintain the workout time variation within each week while doing only four workouts, she should just take one of the five sessions in this Program, divide its time by four, and add the minutes to each of the remaining four workouts.

The time spent in this Program is equivalent to that required to do about 20–25 miles per week of fast PaceWalking™ or running. Now your patient is really getting up there. If he likes this one, he has obviously become hooked on regular exercise. He may also have found that he really likes sports for its own sake, not just for what it does for his mind and body. If that is the case, he may be ready to try doing two or more sports in the same Program. If so, what we call "PaceTraining" is for him (see Chapter 11).

ROADBLOCKS THAT MAY BE ENCOUNTERED, AND HOW TO OVERCOME THEM

There are a series of roadblocks that may be encountered on the road to becoming a regular exerciser. If your patient does meet one or more, she should remember first that she is not alone. Most of us have encountered more than one of these roadblocks, and many people who are now regular exercisers have dealt with them. Here are some suggestions to help overcome them. We are presenting this particular content in the question-and-answer format. The questions are generally those a patient of yours might ask at this point. The answers are offered as experience-based recommendations for what you might say in response.

Suppose Your Patient Says, "I Just Don't Like This."

First, they should hone in on just what it is that they don't like. Is it the regular? Time is the only solution to that problem. Recalling their goal(s), they should try to stick with it, giving themselves a fair shot at overcoming that hurdle. It will help at the beginning if the amount of minutes devoted to ordinary, plain walking is kept low, as provided for in the Getting Started schedule. Until they can manage to get the "regular" built into their lives, they should not try to exercise more than the prescribed three times a week if they are thinking "I don't like this," and mean the number of times they are going out. If what they don't like is walking or whatever the activity is that they chose to start with, they should try another one. And if that doesn't work, then try yet another one. Again, in the next chapter you will see that the range of suitable sports/activities is very broad.

Suppose Your Patient Says "It Hurts."

He should try first to figure out just what hurts. Did he get injured? If so, he should stop working out and come to see you right away. On the other hand, the pain may be the result only of long disuse and accompanying stiffness. The only way to treat this is by stopping for some period of time (or switching to a different activity), not something he really wants to do just as he is trying to get started. Thus, prevention is key. It is important for you to emphasize when starting out, your patient should try to follow all the suggestions you have offered. In summary: *Take it easy at first. Go slowly and not for too long. When starting out, remember that it is far better to underdo it than to overdo it.*

Pain may also be related to a problem with equipment, particularly shoes. A pair of shoes that doesn't fit can cause all sorts of problems, from shin splints to heel and toe blisters. Obviously, your patient doesn't want to go out first thing and spend a lot of money for a good pair of walking, running, or aerobics shoes if she is not really sure she is going to stick with it. But if she has nothing else around the house other than an old pair of sneakers, she may have to do just that. (See Chapter 11 on how to select a good pair of walking/running shoes.) Bad shoes can easily lead to pain and injury, that in turn causes quitting and thus creates a self-fulfilling prophecy. If your patient buys a good pair of shoes and happens not to become a regular exerciser for some other reason, at least he will have a (hopefully) nice-looking and comfortable pair of walking-around shoes.

Suppose Your Patient Says, "I Don't Like Getting up Earlier in the Morning."

First, remember that, even though it is not highly recommended, when starting out on TSTEP, the majority of the minutes can be done on the weekends. And that arrangement can be maintained until he is ready to increase the number of the during-the-week workouts. Second, if he doesn't like working out in the morning, he can consider going out before supper, or a bit after it. Remember, there is plenty of room for flexibility in TSTEP, even with the constraints of consistency and regularity.

Suppose Your Patient Says, Simply, "This Is Just Not Working."

First, she should think of precisely what she means when she says "not working." Does she perhaps mean only "I don't understand it. I've been doing this stuff for three whole months [after a lifetime of living a sedentary lifestyle] and I'm not in tip-top shape yet?" Or are they really saying, "I am not getting immediate gratification from all this work?" There is no easy way to deal with this one. We can only suggest reviewing the material on motivation, goal setting, and the causes of the drive for immediate gratification and how in the long run that drive actually interferes with reaching one's goals. And, remember that when starting from scratch, using the recommended one-step-at-a-time approach, most people will not feel that they are "getting into shape" for at least four months, in many cases six. These things just take time. At any rate, one way or another, they will hopefully complete the first 13 weeks in stride, and be ready to move on to Phase II.

SOME AFTERTHOUGHTS

The Two Kinds of Mental Discipline Required for Success in Regular Exercise

Addressing your patients, you can say that you are of course aware that to achieve success with TSTEP, you need mental discipline. You should be aware that not just one, but two kinds of mental discipline are required. He will need both to stay with regular exercise, to make it a part of his life, to recognize its intrusiveness and deal with it, adapt to it. At the same time, he will also need to be able to do what athletes refer to as "staying within yourself." That's really a part of goal setting.

She must be clear about her goals, and make sure that the goals she decides upon are reasonable ones for her. She should not design a program that requires more effort than she can reasonably make in terms of time and athletic ability, now. Encourage her to explore her limits. She may never know to where they might extend. At the same time, it is essential to recognize one's limitations. Thus, if she gets into a distance-sport like running or cycling, in exploring limits she might find that she can go much further than she thought she could when she started out. At the same time, if a limitation is that she is just naturally slow and would need an awful lot of work to get faster, we advise that she just accept that so that she can continue to explore her limits happily and healthily.

Taking Breaks

Breaks in your patient's exercise program are also important. Having just stressed the importance of routine and consistency, advocating for breaks may sound like a conflicting message. Planned breaks, such as during a short vacation, or after a goal has been reached, help to revitalize both the mind and the body. The break can act as a reward and as a tool to help re-motivate your patient. A short (1–3 weeks) break can be good not only for the mind but also for the body, even though a modest amount of deconditioning may occur. (In most regular exercisers, it will be recovered pretty quickly.) When muscles are stressed (particularly through vigorous-intensity exercise), they require recovery time to 'assimilate the training'—to recover and strengthen from the activity that they have done. The more intensely your patient is exercising, the more benefit he will get from breaks.

Another time in which rest breaks are necessary is during an injury and through illness. As we have mentioned several times, patients should be encouraged to "listen to their bodies"—becoming more observant of the body's messages telling the patient when it is getting injured. Particularly with overuse injuries, the earlier a potential injury can be 'caught' and rested, the shorter the time that the injury will have to be rested. For example, if a patient starts to notice a "nagging" in her calf when she walks briskly, she should try to find an activity that does not aggravate her calf. This may simply be walking at a slower pace, or may involve trying a different sport (such as swimming) for a week. Guided stretching may also help. If these alternatives are not possible, or continue to aggravate her calf, she should stop exercising for a short (1–2 weeks) time, and seek medical attention if the problem does not go away. If she tries to continue exercising through the pain, there could be an injury that worsens, resulting in pain and discomfort during other activities, and a forced break from exercise for a longer (1–2 months) time.

Clearly, during serious illness, patients should not be exercising. During mild illnesses, such as a mild cold or headache, light exercise may be beneficial. Again, our advice is to encourage your patient to listen to her body. If exercising makes her feel better during mild illness, there is no reason to stop. If, however, she feels worse exercising, then a break is indicated.

In addition to planned breaks and illness- or injury-related breaks, other obstacles can lead to unplanned breaks in your patient's exercise program. Help your patient to accept that these breaks are inevitable and are not damaging to the program unless they result in your patient loosing motivation and having difficulty returning to the exercise program. Therefore, ensuring that patients are able to get back to their regular exercise routine after a break—either a planned break or an inevitable, unplanned one—should be a priority for both you and your patient.

Overdoing It

Regular exercise should lead to improved health and fitness, and to feeling good. It should not lead to injury, anxiety, frustration, anger, isolation, and stress. If your patient has it in her to become a good athlete (whether "good" is defined by speed or endurance, by winning, or simply by participation) as well as a regular exerciser, her athletic ability will come out. And then she will find more time for sports. All in good time. In the meantime, as previously noted, she should not overdo it. It's not difficult to get caught up in the exercise fervor when just starting out. One hasn't done anything for a long time. But this time, she convinces himself, she is really going to get into it. And so the first day, she runs five miles, as fast as she can, or she does an hour of high-impact aerobics; or, at age 38, another patient attempts to start weight-lifting at a level close to what he was doing in high school.

The next morning, he and she hurt so much all over that they can barely get out of bed. They may very well (wisely) decide to let the pain subside before they go at it again. But by the time that happens, the fervor may very well have passed. Or, conversely, they may continue at the same level of intensity, deciding to try to work their way through the pain. Commonly, that approach leads to injury. Either way, they are on the road not to success, but to stopping. How much is too much is neither predictable nor quantifiable, nor is it always avoidable. However, for most patients, for the most part, it is better to err on the side of doing a little too little, as long as it is done on a regular basis according to a plan, than to do much too much. Less, especially in intensity, can indeed be more, again as long as it is done on a regular basis. As long as one stays with it, intensity as well as time spent can always be built up. Once again, remind your patients on a regular basis that gradual change leads to permanent changes.

On Knowing When to Stop

And, finally, suppose that your patient has mobilized their motivation, learned the details of training Programs, sports, technique and equipment, got going on TSTEP, and gave it a reasonable and legitimate try. But they found that it just isn't fun. They can't get on a regular schedule. They have tried PaceWalking™, they have tried some of the other sports or activities, they have tried them in combinations. Nothing works. In addition, they find that they are not getting any of the advertised benefits, or, if they are, they feel that the reward does not justify the effort. Then the best thing to do is stop—yes, stop, at least for now. They should not feel guilty about doing so, and it's important that you are able to give your permission to them to do so.

In theory, regular exercise, aerobic or non-aerobic, is good for almost everyone. But maybe it just isn't in the cards for this particular patient at this particular time. Maybe he has not truly mobilized his motivation to get from Stage III

(Planning) to Stage IV (Action). But maybe he never will. That's okay. Maybe he really just doesn't have the time, in a very busy schedule. At least, not now.

Not being a regular exerciser doesn't make one a bad person. There are many good people who are not regular exercisers. If your patient just doesn't like doing it and doesn't feel that they are getting much if anything out of it, they should just stop. For if in this state they try to continue, they will likely become angry and frustrated, and they will certainly raise their level of risk for injury. Yes, your patient does need mental discipline to know when to stop as well as to be able to keep going. And you need the understanding of the whole motivation mobilization process and how we move through the Stages of Change, to be able to give them permission to do so, at the appropriate time.

And then again, maybe six to 12 months from now they will feel differently. They can always give it another go. Maybe looking back on the first time around, they, and you, will note something that they did or didn't do that became an impediment to success, like at the beginning trying too hard to go too far too fast. If that's the case, they can give it another go with a better chance of success. There are plenty of successful regular exercisers who didn't finally get going until they were anywhere from 40 to 80, or even beyond that.

References

1. Jonas S. Triathloning for ordinary mortals. 2nd ed. New York: WW Norton; 2006. Chapter 5, Training basics for triathlon an decathlon; p. 96–125. Chapter 6, Starting from scratch: The basic aerobic fitness program; p. 126–141. Chapter 7, The triathloning for ordinary mortals training program; p. 142–156.
2. Jonas S, Radetsky P. PaceWalking: the balanced way to aerobic health. New York: Crown Publishers; 1988. Chap. 4, The Pace Walking Program; p. 62–81.
3. Jonas S. Take control of your weight. Yonkers (NY): Consumers Reports Books; 1993. Chapter 8, The take control exercise program; p. 133–156.
4. Jonas S. Regular exercise: a handbook for clinical practice. New York: Springer Publishing Co.; 1995. Chapter 6, The regular exerciser's training program; p. 116–150.
5. Walsh C. The Bowerman system. Los Altos (CA): Tafnews Press; 1983. 72 p.

CHAPTER 11

Choosing the Activities, Sport, or Sports

Steven Jonas

INTRODUCTION

As you will have already gathered from the previous chapters, there is a very broad range of lifestyle activities, sports, and other athletic activities to choose from for a regular exercise program. It does not mean simply running or group aerobic exercise/activities (although each of these is a suitable choice for the right person). As we have emphasized throughout the book, both the "lifestyle exercise" approach and the "scheduled leisure time" approach can work, and they do work for different people. Sometimes they both work in conjunction with each other for the same person, done either sequentially throughout the year or in some combination during a given week.

Whatever works for a given patient is what works for *him,* as we have said on more than one occasion. The goal is to get to and maintain, at a minimum, the ACSM minimum of 30 minutes of exercise of moderate intensity at least five times each week. With your guidance, as we demonstrate in this book, there are a variety of routes your patients can and do take to get there. What is fascinating about the whole enterprise, as we too have noted on more than one occasion, is that, for many people—regardless of how they got there—once they get into the habit, they will find it a hard one to kick.

The choices between the lifestyle exercise approach and engaging in scheduled leisure-time workouts—in a sport or other athletic activity, at the gym, at home, on the road, in the park, or what have you—are not mutually exclusive. One can stay with one. One can move from one to the other and back, mixing and matching as they go. In fact, many regular exercisers find that variation of their routines over the course of the year is just what the doctor ordered to keep them fresh over time, to keep them stimulated, and, if an athlete, to work out different muscle groups at different times of the year. For example, one of us, a long-time triathlete and downhill skier, engages in his swim-bike-run training program from mid-March to mid-October and then switches to weight-training and body conditioning to prepare for ski season, as well as during the winter to, as he ages, build up muscle strength for the next year's triathlon season. He has been doing this for over 25 years.

LIFESTYLE EXERCISE: SOME OF THE POPULAR CHOICES

Introduction

Lifestyle exercise is an opportunity for your patient to achieve most of the general health benefits of exercise (1, 2, 3) through physical activity of moderate intensity. Your patient does this by doing at a higher level the daily physical activities that he ordinarily does at a fairly low level, and by introducing physical activity into one's daily routine. For example, you may advise your patient to begin his program of regular exercise by taking the stairs at work instead of waiting for the elevator or escalator. For very deconditioned or elderly patients, light activity will provide general health benefits and an introduction to higher-intensity physical activity. (See Three-Minute Drill 11-1.)

Intensity

But how can you explain to your patient how intense "moderate" is? If the activity, such as walking, is intense enough that your patient can still talk but cannot sing, then she is exercising at a moderate level (see also Table 8.3). More precisely, a brisk walk is between 3 mph and 4 mph, or approximately 3–5 metabolic equivalents (METs) (see Table 8.3). This can be described to patients as "somewhere between a comfortable pedestrian stroll and a rush to keep an appointment."

Furthermore, moderate-intensity exercise is done at a pace that can be maintained comfortably for at least 45 minutes.

These examples refer to walking as the mode of physical activity, as it is the most common form of exercise and, for many, the easiest form to fit into their normal daily routine. However, other forms of exercise, such as biking, swimming, or going to the gym are also excellent ways for patients to exercise at a moderate-intensity level. (See Chapter 8, pp. 99–133, for recommendations on additional types of exercise.)

THREE-MINUTE DRILL, 11 – 1

Some Advantages of Lifestyle Exercise:

- Less time-intrusive than scheduled leisure-time exercise
- Can seem less intimidating to individuals who are nervous about "exercising," or who do not think of themselves as "athletes"
- Environmentally friendly
- Provides the majority of the general health benefits of physical activity
- Provides baseline level of fitness on which to build to more vigorous exercise
- Can enable the person to achieve the recommended levels for regular exercise
- Supports behavior change models advocating for small change
- Sets a good example for colleagues (may motivate them to join you)

Advantages of the Lifestyle Exercise Approach and Choices

For many average, sedentary persons, lifestyle exercise can be sufficient to raise their energy expenditure level to the point where they are no longer considered sedentary. As specified in the ACSM/AHA recommendations (4), more vigorous activity confers greater benefits and begins to positively impact on physical fitness.

The lifestyle exercise approach has many advantages. Lifestyle exercise is usually not as time-intrusive as scheduled leisure-time exercise. The lifestyle exercises often replace with greater physical activity time spent passively. For example, commuters who use public transportation to get to work could get off the train or the bus a stop early, which may allow for a 10-minute walk to their workplace. Similarly, parking at the back of a parking lot exchanges the time spent walking for the time spent circling the lot looking for a closer spot. By engaging in these simple activities, your patients can reach their goal of 30 minutes per day five days per week, through the accumulation of three such lifestyle activities, each of 10 minutes in duration. The choice is extensive (Three-Minute Drill 11-2).

Lifestyle exercise can also improve your patient's strength and flexibility, from such activities as engaging in gentle stretching while speaking on the

THREE-MINUTE DRILL, 11 – 2

Some Ways to be More Active Every Day:

- Incorporate walking into daily commute. In an urban setting, get off the bus or train one stop earlier and walk.
- Take the stairs instead of the elevator or escalator.
- Park at the back of the lot and walk.
- Engage gardening.
- Use a push hand or mechanical lawn mower.
- Shovel your sidewalk.
- Rake the leaves instead of using a mechanical blower.
- Organize a "walking school bus," rather than driving to school.
- Plan a walking meeting at work, rather than sitting around the table.
- Walk with your kids to a neighborhood park, rather than watching TV with them.
- Bike to work or to other activities.
- Do static exercises (lunges, heel raises, etc) while talking on the phone.
- Walk to your local grocery store (fill a backpack), use soup cans to do bicep/tricep curls on the walk home.
- When waiting for a flight, walk the halls of the airport rather than sitting in the waiting room.
- Stretch while waiting for the bus.
- Take regular stretch breaks during your work day.

phone to pushing a lawn mower around the yard rather than riding on one. The intermittent nature of lifestyle exercise, such as adding stair climbing periodically throughout the day, is supported by the exercise recommendations to *accumulate* 30 minutes of moderate physical activity most, if not all days of the week. The ACSM guidelines suggest that each bout of exercise should be approximately 10 minutes in duration to be counted towards the 30-minute goal (4).

Increasing Physical Activity

Throughout this book we have chosen to use the word *exercise* to represent both scheduled leisure-time exercise and moderate physical activity undertaken in the course of the day intense enough to generate general health benefits. Many of your patients may express antipathy to the perceived challenges and pain of regular exercise, thinking that it can be only of the scheduled leisure-time type, whether a sport or other athletic activity such as "going to the gym." Explaining the benefits of moderate physical activity that does not necessarily require sweating, feeling pain, changing clothes, becoming out of breath, or spending money for equipment may very well significantly help your patients in mobilizing their motivation for regular exercise.

Because it is not seen nearly as demanding, or life-changing, or even threatening in one way or another as trying to engage in regularly scheduled leisure-time exercise, recommending lifestyle exercise is a great way to help your patients mobilize their motivation to become more active. ("What, me, I should try to become an athlete? Who are you kidding?") Many folks get into regular exercise through the lifestyle approach and then switch over to the scheduled leisure-time approach. But many others start with the lifestyle approach and stay with it indefinitely. As we have noted more than once, the benefits of increased physical activity are incremental, *i.e.,* the more you do, the higher the resultant level of fitness. The simple message for your patients is, "Something is better than nothing, and more is better than less."

The physiologic benefits of gradually increasing physical activity support the processes of mobilizing motivation and beginning to undertake the behavior changes discussed in Chapters 4–6. Small initial changes in behavior can lead to initial small successes that can gradually increase feelings of self-efficacy ("Yes, I can do this when I put my mind to it"). Then that boost in self-confidence leads to undertaking the next small change, and so on and so forth. These successive small changes then lead to larger and sustained lifestyle changes. As we have said on more than one occasion: "gradual change leads to permanent changes." An easy way to start on the pathway of gradual change is to engage in the lifestyle exercise approach.

Becoming a *regular* lifestyle exerciser means continuously looking for opportunities to add physical activity to everyday activities. Both setting aside the time for regular leisure-time scheduled activity and engaging in regular lifestyle exercise require mindfulness and planning. While awareness and planning are necessary in order to increase one's level of physical activity, convenience can also be an important factor in doing so. Convenience is an important plus for the lifestyle approach. This is where the "built environment" becomes a factor. For example, the availability of safe routes and adequate sidewalks or pathways to walk to school or to work is an important element for many that will determine how much lifestyle exercise they can introduce into their daily routine. The built environment is also an important factor in determining the level of the baseline activity within a community. Urbanites routinely walk more than suburbanites and are six pounds lighter than their counterparts who more readily use cars even to cover short distances.

Creating a baseline of daily physical activity establishes a foundation on which your patients can build to engage in more regular exercise. It is possible, for instance, to move from lifestyle exercise to scheduled exercise, should one want to do so, by using a "counting pedometer" (that is, one that counts steps taken) or other similar device to record activity. Wearing the pedometer through a day of work may reveal that your patient has taken 3,000 to 5,000 steps. If the daily goal is 10,000 steps, then the patient would most likely need to set aside scheduled exercise time to complete the daily goal.

Pedometers are an easily accessible and inexpensive way to measure physical activity throughout the day. Commonly, pedometers measure the numbers of steps, distance, and calories, though the most accurate and important measure is simply the number of steps per day. More sophisticated devices distinguish between simple movement at low intensity from moderate-intensity brisk walking at a rate of at least 120 steps per minute, or continuous movement for at least 10 minutes.

Using the Pedometer

A baseline of several thousand steps per day will usually be achieved through the simple activities of daily living. Additional steps are generally accrued on the average at 2,000 steps to the mile. National programs advocating 10,000 steps per day are consistent with the recommended 30 minutes of moderate-intensity daily activity, because sessions of additional walking are necessary to achieve this goal. (See Table 11.1 for gradations of activity measured in steps/day.)

Interestingly, pedometers may be used to measure both lifestyle exercise through daily activities as well as structured exercise. As an example, your patient with a goal of 10,000 steps may achieve 7,500 steps through the course of their day, including a brief lunchtime walk and taking the stairs instead of the elevator. After work they may then complete the goal with a planned 2,500-step walk around the neighborhood.

As covered in Chapters 4–6 on motivation and the recommended progression of the exercise prescription in Chapter 8, to best engage your patients it is important to set short-term achievable goals. Table 11.2 presents a program to

TABLE 11.1 Steps/Day Physical Activity Index for Adults

Steps/Day	Physical Activity Level
<5,000	Sedentary
5,000–7,499	Low Active
7,500–9,999	Somewhat Active
10,000–12,499	Active
>12,500	Highly Active

Source: Tudor-Locke C, Bassett DR Jr. How many steps/day are enough? preliminary pedometer indices for public health. Sports Med. 2004 Mon; 34(1):1–8.

establish a baseline of daily step counts, and then each week to add 500 steps/day. The additional steps done at a moderately intense pace of 120 steps per minute will take less than 5 minutes to complete.

Your encouragement to adopt a more active lifestyle is supported by the gradually developing societal change towards encouraging more environmentally friendly physical activities of daily living. A shift towards raking the lawn rather than using a mechanical blower, or shoveling snow (that is, if one is sure that one has no known risk factors for a heart attack) rather than using a snow blower, are both environmentally sound practices and ways to be more active. You may recommend that even in the midst of a leisure activity, golf for instance, your patients walk the course (or part of the course) rather than ride

TABLE 11.2 Determining Baseline Steps/Day and Increasing Steps/Day

Phase	Instructions
Step 1: Baseline steps/day	Keep track of steps/day over a typical 4–7 period.
Step 2: Benchmark	Make your daily step count for week #1 the highest daily steps/day count that was achieved in the baseline (Step 1) phase
Step 3: Build	After week #1, try to add 500 steps/day each week until the goal is met.

Source: Le Masurier G. Walkee talkee: answers to pedometer FAQs [Internet]. ACSM Fit Society®. [c2005; cited 2008 Jun 22]. 2 p. Available from: http://www.acsm.org/AM/Template.cfm?Section=ACSM_Fit_Society_Page&TPLID=2&TPPID=413&TEMPLATE=/TaggedPage/TaggedPageDisplay.cfm&CONTENTID=4393

a golf cart. You might even have the temerity to suggest that when walking the course, they carry their bag rather than wheel it on a cart!

Conclusion

For many patients, a combination of lifestyle/scheduled leisure-time exercise prescription may reasonably include a blend of 30 minutes of accumulated moderate physical activity most, if not every day of the week, with several sessions of exercise classes or more vigorous, planned regular exercise. Now let us turn to a consideration of the sports and other athletic activities that can be used in the scheduled leisure-time approach.

THE SPORTS AND ATHLETIC ACTIVITIES THAT CAN BE USED FOR LEISURE-TIME SCHEDULED EXERCISE

Principles

If your patient is considering leisure-time scheduled exercise, it is both important and useful for him to understand that the choice of sports and other athletic activities (such as using an elliptical trainer, treadmill, rowing machine, or exercise bicycle at home or at the gym) is very extensive. As we have noted, it is not just walking/running or group aerobic exercise/activities anymore. In this section we'll review the list of some of the more popular ones, with the understanding that there are still others not included. For patients who would like to do scheduled exercise, it is likely that they will be able to find at least one sport or athletic activity that they will like, or come to like over time. Many people engage in more than one, either at the same time or over the course of the calendar year.

Patience is important here. Again, the most important part of this whole enterprise is the mobilization of motivation and the subsequent setting of goals. Once your patient has done that, finding the appropriate activity can be considered commentary. If they don't know in advance what they would like to do, trial and error is a method for choosing that can work very well. They just shouldn't load up on expensive equipment (see Chapter 12) before they are sure that they like the sport they are buying the equipment for. There are enough costly not-purpose-designed dust-collectors/clothes-racks that have accumulated in enough basements and spare bedrooms around the country.

For those patients who like to work out in groups, there are many choices, including (but not limited to), a wide variety of group dance classes (formerly called "aerobic dance") and other exercise/activities such as stepping; group water exercise (especially useful for overweight patients); exercise kickboxing/ martial arts classes; Pilates; yoga; group strength, stretching and core conditioning classes; and group indoor exercise machine (bicycles, treadmills, elliptical trainers, etc.) classes.

We would like to re-emphasize that it is very important for both you and your patients to understand that it's different strokes for different folks when it comes to choosing a sport or other athletic activity. Once again, there is no one sport that is ideal for everyone. There is no one sport that is better than any of the others. One size does **not** fit all. If regularity is to be maintained, it is of vital importance for each person to choose what works for her, to choose for her activity/sport what she likes, or feels she can learn to like.

This principle can be summed up in the sentence: "The **best** exercise for you is the exercise that's best for **you**." It may sound like a no-brainer to also say that the best sport for you is the one that is best for you. But that's the truth, and it is worthwhile repeating, both for yourself and for your patients. When your patient gets to the point of engaging in a sport, one of the keys to success is picking the one that is right for him, one he is comfortable with, can do, that will be fun for him—if not at first, then eventually.

When one is considering engaging in a sport or sports, a very important point is that there clearly are choices. Your patient should use them. And if she makes the wrong choice the first time around, she should be encouraged not to simply give up. She should be encouraged try another sport or two. Given the very broad range of sports available, most folks are able to find something that is both suitable and fun for them.

The Sports

Turning now to a consideration of the available sports, first they can be grouped by type.

1. *Skill/Non-Skill*

    The list of the skill sports useful for a regular exercise program begins with the well-known ones that require some level of hand-eye coordination: tennis (singles tennis is clearly an aerobic sport), any of the other racquet sports played as singles, handball, squash, competitive badminton (never seen competitive badminton? It can be brutal), and golf (yes, golf—if one carries or even wheels one's bag around the 18 holes and does not use the golf cart at all—does provide a very good walking workout). Other skill sports that can be used as part of a regular exercise program for at least part of the year in various parts of the country include swimming (which even at slow speeds does require a modicum of skill), kayaking, in-line roller skating (becoming increasingly popular), weight-lifting and other types of resistance training, cross-country skiing (one of the most aerobic sports, actually, and it can be done both outdoors and indoors on a machine), ice-skating, snow-shoeing (also highly aerobic and it does require some skill to stay up), and even downhill skiing and riding (if you do either vigorously enough, with few stops on each run and short lift lines).

    The non-skill set includes the distance-sports done at the non-competitive level, such as fast walking, what we call PaceWalking™, (see

Chapter 12), and, yes, there is of course race-walking (actually a skill sport with its own racing circuit—both it and fast walking can be used in long-distance road races such as marathons), jogging/running (as we have noted elsewhere, the famous physician guru of running, Dr. George Sheehan once famously said "the difference between a jogger and a runner is a race entry blank"), cycling, rowing, and hiking. The distance-sports become skill sports when one starts to speed up and especially if one gets into racing (see below).

2. *Outdoor/Indoor*

Many of the sports listed above can be done both outdoors and indoors, while others are exclusive to one arena or the other. It is important to note that for the sports that can be done in both settings, like walking/running and cycling, some folks are happy doing it in either location. However, for others, jogging on a treadmill with the headset on or the TV going is just great, but jogging outside, with the air pollution, the traffic and the traffic noise—are you kidding? Then there are the cyclists for whom riding in the fresh air and the bright sun is just ticket, while they would never ever ride on what for them would be a totally boring exercycle.

PaceWalking™ and jogging/running can be done on the treadmill, on indoor and outdoor tracks, on the streets and roads (if one is careful), in city parks, on country and country park trails. Swimming can be done in indoor pools (at the "Y," at certain gyms) and in open water, lake or ocean, even rivers and streams that do not have strong currents. Cycling can be done indoors on an exercycle or on a regular bicycle mounted on what's called an indoor trainer, and outdoors on the road or trail (the latter with a suitable bicycle). Rowing can be done indoors on a machine or on the water in a scull or a rowboat.

The most commonly engaged in indoor athletic activities are those done at the gym. As noted above, these include weight-training of one sort or another, using a variety of machines and/or free weights or some combination of both. There are group aerobic exercise/activities and all of its variations, stepping, kick-boxing, and other martial arts exercises. Then there is the increasing number of variations on the elliptical trainer, the stair climbers, the arm cycles, and similar gadgets. The number of available machines seems to multiply every year. You can do many of these activities at home as well, doing your workout along with music tapes, a video, a computer program, or one of the exercise programs that appear throughout the day on television (check your local listings). There are some folks who are lucky enough to have a set of gym equipment in their basements or attics, and actually use them on a regular basis, other than as clothes-drying racks.

3. *Team*

Finally, there are the team sports (which could also be included under the skill sports), several of which can be done aerobically or at a pace quick enough to enable the breaking of a sweat and an increase in the breathing rate. Included on this list are soccer football, field hockey, lacrosse, ice hockey, two-person volleyball, and full-court basketball.

We are sure that we have forgotten to mention at least a few of the sports that can be used for at least a part of a scheduled exercise program. If you have a suggestion, please send it to us c/o the publications office at ACSM (address on the copyright page) and we will be sure to include it in the next edition of this book.

PACETRAINING

One does not have to limit oneself to doing just one sport at a time. There are many advantages to "cross-training," that is, doing two or more sports concurrently in a regular program. Because we consider PaceWalking™ (described in some detail in the next chapter) to be the "FAST," the Foundation Aerobic SporT, the authors' term for cross-training is "PaceTraining."

Introduction

PaceTraining is working out in two or more sports on a regular basis in the same program, for health, fitness, and fun. As noted, PaceTraining is an adaptation of "cross-training," a workout system originally developed by and for single sport racers who wanted to achieve and maintain a high level of aerobic fitness while reducing their overuse injury risk in their racing sport. Thus, we consider cross-training to be for racers, while PaceTraining is for any regular exerciser. PaceTraining focuses on the enjoyment of sports in general, not speed or skill in any particular sport.

The theory of PaceTraining recognizes that any aerobic exercise improves your heart's ability to do work over time, that is, its fitness level. When you are exercising, your heart doesn't "know" which sport you are doing. However, it does respond to the call upon it to work harder. Thus, in a PaceTraining program in which you are working aerobically, your aerobic fitness will improve regardless of how many aerobic sports you include in it. PaceTraining can be used by folks exercising on a non-aerobic basis as well, and confers many of the same advantages it does to aerobically-exercising athletes. For a Pace-Training program, your patient simply chooses the two or more sports that she wants to do. Likely being on Phase III or IV of the STEP, one might ride the bike (indoors or outdoors) twice a week, swim once, and PaceWalk twice. The sports can be mixed and matched as one pleases.

The Major Advantages of PaceTraining

PaceTraining has five major advantages over single-sport training:

1. By building psychological and physical variety into training, the boredom potential of regular exercise will be significantly reduced.
2. By exercising and developing two or more major muscle groups at the same time, overall muscle balance will be promoted.
3. The risk of both intrinsic and extrinsic injury (see Chapter 7) that accompanies every sport to a greater or lesser extent will be reduced, compared with what that risk would be if one did just one of the sports exclusively.
4. Exercising aerobically in a PaceTraining program will build up cardiovascular fitness without risking overuse or strain of any one major muscle group.
5. Exercising aerobically in a PaceTraining program will improve the ability of all the muscles in your body to use the oxygen the blood supplies to them.

On this last point, each major health and fitness sport focuses on one major group of muscles. Running uses primarily the hamstrings and the calf muscles, while also involving the quadriceps and the lower back. In PaceWalking™ your leg muscles are used more, of course, but the hip and lower back muscles are more involved than they are in running. With its vigorous arm-swing (see Chapter 12) PaceWalking™ also exercises the muscles of the shoulders and upper back. Bicycling relies mainly on the lower back muscles and quads, and the calves as well, if bike shoe cleats are used (see Chapter 12) and a pull-up is incorporated into the pedal stroke. Swimming free style is primarily an upper-body sport, with some leg involvement in the flutter kick. If one is going to use only one of the major workout sports for TSTEP, only PaceWalking™, weight-training, and aerobic dance (and its variants) will provide a relatively complete body workout each time. PaceTraining thus confers many advantages.

While PaceTraining is designed to be fun while reducing your injury risk, it is not magic and it is not painless. There simply are no miraculous, "one-minute," or "five-minute," or "12-minute" or "two-week" solutions for becoming healthy and fit through exercise. To get the many benefits of exercise, both time and work are needed. PaceTraining requires commitment, just like any of TSTEP Phases. It requires mental discipline, consistency, and regularity. But it can make regular exercise more fun and more beneficial for your patients.

THE PLACE OF THE RACE

As noted above, the late, great cardiologist and 1970s guru of running, Dr. George Sheehan, once said "the difference between a jogger and a runner is a race entry blank." And so the three-times-a-week jogger, who never goes more than three miles at a time around the high school track, can explore her limits—become a runner, entering that first five-kilometer ("5k," 3.1 mile) local road race, then going for five miles, then doing her first 10k (and what an achievement, going 6.2 miles in, let us say, 67 minutes, without stopping!).

And later still, marathon thoughts may start creeping into her mind. You know—marathoning—the sport suitable only for masochists. But she ventures out to try a half-marathon, and when that goes well, the course is determined. However, she never would have gotten there if she had not explored her limits, with your help.

On the other hand, it is important to note, her limit may have been reached when she completed that first 10k. And that would be fine. For someone who had previously always circled around the parking lot in her car at the mall for ten minutes in order to pick up a parking spot as close as possible to the main entrance, completing a 10k would be some achievement, wouldn't it? You can offer important assistance in that case, too.

And, of course, for many of your patients, no kind of racing is on the agenda, and should not be. Racing is certainly not for everyone, and there are certainly many healthy, fit, regular exercisers who will never set foot on a racecourse. And that's just fine, too. Although, for one of us, racing (at a slow pace, mind you) became a major part of his life, starting at middle age, it certainly doesn't work for everyone. Again, you can be of great help in helping each patient to define success in terms that suit them.

For those who may be interested in racing, there are a variety of places where race locations, times, and dates can be found. They include local running, cycling, and other sports equipment stores, local health and fitness clubs, and local, state, regional, and national racing clubs and associations for running, cycling, swimming, and triathlon that can be located through the above-named facilities, or by doing a search on the Web. If one starts out with running or swimming, equipment needs are very modest (see the next chapter for a more detailed discussion of equipment).

There is a very long list of publications concerned with racing of various types that can be located on the Web. This is not the place to review the many details with which one can become concerned if one gets into the activity. However, there are a few words of advice for the racing beginner which you might find useful to share. First, the first goal for racing should be to see if your patient likes doing it or not. Racing, as we have said, is not for everyone. Second, while one explores one's limits, and we have said this on a number of occasions, one should recognize one's limitations. For short running and swimming races, one needs speed in order to participate; for longer races, especially in running and multi-sport (triathlon and duathlon), one does not. Distance racing can be enjoyed by just about anyone who determines that they can go the distance as long as they stay at a comfortable speed and don't mind how long they take to get to the finish line. Most distance-race courses will be kept open until most, if not all of the entrants cross the finish line, regardless of how long it takes them.

Third, one should use the first few races of any kind to start learning about the logistics of the particular kind of event one enters. For running distance races, it is pretty simple. One shows up at the starting area allowing enough time to get themselves and their stuff organized, warm up a bit, and then when the starting gun goes off, off one goes. For swimming races, it is rather more complicated, what with having to get to the pool, change clothing, get in warm-ups if permitted, and so on and so forth. Particularly when starting out in the activity, one should always allow more time rather than less to get to the event and prepare for it. For multi-sport racing, the logistics can appear to be fairly complex for the beginner, what with doing two (duathlon: run-bike-run) or three (triathlon: swim-bike-run) sports in succession. For the first-timer, it will be very helpful to get a book on the subject either from the library or by bookstore, or have an experienced friend who can be a guide, or go to an introductory class or two organized by a local triathlon club or coaching concern.

A final word on training and racing: Some people race because they train. They have become regular exercisers in one or more sports, discover that they are training enough to enable them to comfortably complete in races at one distance or another, at speeds they can manage, and that they have fun doing so—so they race. Others train because they race, or rather because they want to race. In other words, it is the racing that keeps them going in their training programs. If they didn't race, they would not train or at least wouldn't train as much as they do. Either approach is fine. But in terms of organizing and following through on one's training program(s), it does help to know which group one is in.

And with these words, we can say, getting to the starting line can be great fun and crossing the finish line can be even more fun.

References

1. Haskell WL, Minn LI, Pate RR, Powell KE, Blair SN, Franklin BA, Macera, CA, Health GW, Thompson PD, Bauman A. Physical activity and public health: updated recommendations from the American College of Sports Medicine and the American Heart Association. Med Sci Sports Exer. 2007 August;39(8):1423–34.
2. U.S. Department of Health and Human Services. Physical activity and health: a report of the Surgeon General. Atlanta (GA): U.S. Department of Health and Human Services, Centers for Disease Control and Prevention, and National Center for Chronic Disease Prevention and Health Promotion; 1996. 278 p.
3. American College of Sports Medicine. Position stand: the recommended quantity and quality of exercise for developing and maintaining cardiorespiratory and muscular fitness and flexibility in healthy adults. Med Sci Sports Exerc. 1998 June;30(6):975–91.
4. Haskell WH, Lee IM, Pate RR, Powell KE, Blair SN, Franklin BA, Macera CA, Heath GW, Thompson PD, Bauman A. Physical activity and public health: updated recommendations for adults from the American College of Sports Medicine and the American Heart Association. Circulation. 2007 August;116(9):1081–93.

CHAPTER 12

Technique and Equipment

Steven Jonas

INTRODUCTION

For The Scheduled Training Exercise Program (TSTEP), good technique is important for any of the sports in which your patient may engage. This is true whether the sport is simple, like running, or somewhat complex, like swimming. However, to enjoy any of the sports or activities useful for regular exercise, one does not have to have *great* technique. No one needs to become especially focused on technique, unless it becomes apparent that he has the potential to become competitive in his chosen sport, and wants to do that. Becoming a technique fanatic can take away from the fun and enjoyment of what is a recreational activity for most regular exercisers, and might even get in the way of staying with it. On the equipment side, while for the sports that require specialized equipment, it should be of good quality, fortunately, one does not need expensive equipment for most of the sports suitable for exercising regularly. Nor is it healthful to become an equipment fanatic, buying various pieces of it just to have them, rather than to make good use of them.

It is a good idea to resist perfectionism as we strive to reach the suitable, realistic goals in health promotion that we have set for ourselves. "We can never be perfect; we can always get better" is a useful standard for the regular exerciser. Thus, *some* time spent on technique is time well spent. A *reasonable* amount of money spent for decent, safe equipment is money well spent. Good technique and equipment will make doing one's chosen sport(s) comfortable and more fun.*

Does good technique have utility if one is not a competitive athlete? Certainly. Take swimming as an example. Let's say you naturally do what, in the New York City region at any rate, is called the "Coney Island Crawl": head always out of the water, moving from side to side with each stroke, arms flailing away, much splash production. Unless you are in extraordinarily good

---

*Note to the reader: This chapter in particular is for the most part voiced as if it were directly addressing the patient, not the professional reader, just as the health professional would be doing in practice.

shape, you will get tired very quickly. While the exercise will most likely be aerobic, if you cannot finish your workout, or, more seriously, if you get into trouble in the water or suffer an injury, your health and fitness will not be served. In running, landing properly on the heel (the best technique for recreational running) can reduce the pounding that normally accompanies that sport, reducing injury risk. In cycling, learning proper gear selection is very important.

In this chapter, we offer some brief recommendations on technique for some of the more popular activities and sports used for regular exercise. Our primary focus is on the one many people will use as their first sport, if they have not exercised regularly before (and, in some cases, even if they have and are starting out once again): PaceWalking™. For three of the other sports commonly used by regular exercisers, a few of the high points on technique are presented. For details on any of them, we suggest that you consult one or more of any number of specialized single-sport books that are available.

While PaceWalking™ is emphasized here, remember, the right sport for *you* is the sport that's *right* for you: one that's fun, that you can do comfortably with some proficiency, one in which you can reach your desired intensity level for the desired amount of time. In this chapter we will also cover the bare basics of equipment for several of the sports commonly used in a regular exercise program. Again, you are referred to one or more of the sport-specific books for details, much more details.

WALKING

Introduction

The late, great George Sheehan, M.D., from the mid-1970s until his untimely death in 1993 was widely known as the "guru" of running for health and fitness. In 1986, after having had for some years made disparaging remarks about walking, Dr. Sheehan pronounced it "the best exercise of all" (1). Exactly 200 years earlier, in 1786, Thomas Jefferson noted (2, p. 16):

"No one knows, till he tries, how easily a habit of walking is acquired. A person who never walked 3 miles will in the course of a month become able to walk 15 or 20 [!] without fatigue. I have known some great walkers and never knew or heard of one who was not healthy and long-lived."

One might question his analysis of cause and effect in this case, but certainly not his enthusiasm for walking.

Ordinary walking is that motion of the body used by everyone who is physically able as the primary means of getting around. It is one of those activities we all do with little if any consciousness of the motion. The most important biomechanical characteristic of walking is that one foot is always in contact with the ground. That is what differentiates walking from running. In running, you are air-borne for at least an instant between each step.

As to its intensity potential, walking for exercise has become increasingly popular over the years. Increasingly one sees statements like, "walking is as good for fitness as running is," or "walking burns about the same number of calories as running does." At the same time, you might have read something like "well, walking is OK, but you have to walk twice as long as you need to run in order to achieve the same benefit." As the first two quotes imply, any sport can be the aerobic equivalent of any other, *if* it is done intensively enough to raise your heart rate to the same level achieved with any of the other sports. If not, then, yes, you may need to spend up to twice as much time to achieve the same result. *It is intensity and heart rate, indicating a given muscle oxygen uptake level, that count, not the particular sport or activity being done.*

PaceWalking™
THE BASICS

We have used the term "PaceWalking™" throughout this book. It is simply walking fast using a defined technique that differs from that of ordinary walking (3, 4). Fast walking also goes by a wide variety of other names: "exercise walking," "fitness walking," "health walking," "power walking," "aerobic walking," "sportwalking." Functionally, PaceWalking™ is walking for sport, exercise, and health, done at your own pace. As noted, it may be done aerobically and non-aerobically. *Done at the same level of intensity for the same amount of time,* PaceWalking™ will do for your body and your mind what any of the other exercise sports will do.

INTRODUCTION TO THE TECHNIQUE

PaceWalking™ is simple to do. You walk fast with a purposeful stride of medium length. With each stride, you land on your heel, roll forward along the outside of your foot, and push off from your toes into the next stride. With each stride, be sure that one foot is always on the ground. Always having at least one foot in contact with the ground is what makes PaceWalking™ walking, and what makes it a rather more gentle sport than running. The PaceWalker tries to be relaxed, standing comfortably straight, not rigidly so, head up, shoulders relaxed and dropped. Muscle tension just leads to pain. Also, having the upper body nice and loose makes it easier to develop a smooth, rhythmic, comfortable, arm swing. To achieve a higher level of intensity, unlike in running, the arm motion is as important as the leg motion. Most people find it impossible to walk fast enough to get their heart rate up without a determined and constant rhythmic swing of the arms.

Your arm swing should be forward and back, in the direction you are moving. Your elbows should be comfortably bent. If you keep them straight, like some fast walkers do, you will end up pooling fluid in your hands. You should not move your arms across your chest. Although that may look good and feel vigorous, it hinders your forward momentum, and may lead to body imbalance and possible injury. Obviously, your left arm should go forward with your right leg, and vice versa. Your fingers should be closed lightly, your fists never clenched. Swinging your arm forward, your hand should reach about to upper chest level. On the swing back, you should stop when you feel your back shoulder muscles gently but firmly stretching. It is the combination of leg stride and arm swing that provides PaceWalking™ with one of the advantages it has over most of the other major distance sports. That is, Pace-Walking™ exercises two, not just one of the major muscle groups.

"PACE" AS SPEED

As in all forward-motion sports, the speed you can eventually reach in Pace-Walking™ is the product of natural ability, practice, and level of fitness. When you begin, you will probably be doing the mile in about 15 to 18 minutes. (The average pace for ordinary walking is about 20 minutes per mile.) With some practice, you can get down to 13–14 minutes per mile; 11–12 minutes per mile is a good clip in PaceWalking™.

PACEWALKING™: THE FOUNDATION AEROBIC SPORT; FAST

Finally, PaceWalking™ is truly the FAST exercise. How, you might ask, can a sport that's intrinsically slow compared with the other forward-motion sports be fast? Well, it's not that it's fast, but rather that it's "The FAST," the foundation on which you can build a basic level of fitness from which you can then go on to do other sports. You will gradually, easily, but steadily work yourself into shape. Your injury risk will be low. Your workouts will be pleasant, with little pain. Once you have established your fitness base with PaceWalking™, you will find that any of the other regular exercise sports (or two or more of them in a PaceTraining program) can come very easily to you, if you want it to.

THE OTHER POPULAR DISTANCE SPORTS FOR REGULAR EXERCISE

In this section we will briefly review some aspects of technique for three of the other popular distance sports that you can do in TSTEP. It should be noted that these sports can be done both indoors and outdoors.

Running

Running is familiar to just about everyone. It is one of the most popular sports for regular exercise, although fast walking is gradually catching up. For most people, running is aerobic at all but the slowest of speeds. Basic running technique is simple. A former national-class hurdler once described as "left, right, left, right." Well it's not quite *that* simple, but it's close. As in PaceWalking™, it is important to keep your body relaxed, back comfortably but not rigidly straight, shoulders dropped, elbows comfortably bent, fingers lightly closed (fists not clenched). For the foot strike, as in PaceWalking™, you land on your heel, not the sole or ball of your foot. You roll forward along the outside edge of the foot, and then spring forward off the ball of your foot into the next stride. Just as in PaceWalking™, you should aim for balance, rhythm, and smoothness.

Cycling

Outdoor cycling is most enjoyable, but if you want it to be aerobic, you need to work fairly hard to make it so. On a bicycle, it is very easy to glide along at 8–10 miles per hour. But most people need to ride at least 13–15 miles per hour to achieve and maintain an aerobic heart rate. And that takes some effort. Top-form outdoor cycling technique is complex. It takes instruction, time, and practice to learn. However, there are a few simple principles which will serve to get you started safely and help you to ride effectively and efficiently.

Most important is "cadence," the cyclists' term for pedal revolutions per minute (rpm). The most efficient way to bike is using a relatively high cadence in a relatively low gear. For beginners, that means pedaling in the 60–70 rpm range. With experience, you will easily be able to work up to the 80–90 rpm range, called "spinning." At the other end of the spectrum, except when going up a really steep hill, pedaling slowly in a high gear, below 50 rpm, pushing a heavy load with your legs, is an invitation to knee problems. You should try to avoid it.

In terms of position, your upper body should be relaxed. Pain across your upper back is the primary result of scrunching up your shoulders. Helping to absorb road shock, your elbows should be comfortably bent. There are two primary hand positions on the bike that has curved handle bars: on the hoods that cover the brake handles, and on the "drops," that is the lower curved parts. As your speed increases on a bike, you spend an increasing amount of your energy just moving air out of your way. Thus the lower down you get over the handlebars on a road bike, the more efficiently you will be riding. Hand position on a mountain bike is simple (unless you are riding a racing model): out on the ends of the bars, where the grips are.

As for gear-shifting, on both the mountain and the road bike, you will notice that the pedals are attached to two or three toothed "chain rings" and from which the chain runs back to six to ten smaller "cogs" on the right side of the rear wheel hub. It is the particular combination of front and rear rings around which the chain is looped that determines the "gear" the bike is in at any one time. A higher, harder gear is one in which the chain is on a large ring up front and a small one at the back. Conversely, the combination of a smaller chain ring up front and a relatively larger cog at the back produces a lower, easier, gear. The lower gears are used when going up hill, the medium ones when on the flat, and the higher ones when going downhill. Gear shift levers come in a variety of locations and combinations on the bike. Their correct use is best learned from an experienced cyclist friend or cycle-shop staffer.

Swimming

As long as you feel psychologically comfortable in the water, swimming is a very comfortable sport physically. The water supports most of your weight. There is none of the pounding, twisting, and jarring that is associated with running. Swimming can be a good exercise for very heavy people to start out with. The water supports a great deal of the body's weight, easing the strain on muscles, joints, and heart. Further, when they first start exercising, some heavy people may be shy about "appearing in public." The water can provide a convenient screen.

Good swimming technique is somewhat complex and takes some time and practice to learn. Smoothness and rhythm are absolutely essential in this sport. So is proper breathing, arm position through the stroke, and leg position. Few people can learn to swim safely and efficiently on their own, without instruction. If you don't know how to swim but want to try it, find a local "Y" or swim club that offers lessons. There is a certain amount of fear to overcome, and it is very easy to get into bad habits without knowing it. Personal instruction can really help in dealing with these problems, as well as with the technical aspects of the sport.

WEIGHT TRAINING

As noted, the ACSM recommends that all adults engage in weight training (also known as resistance training) on a regular basis, as part of their program of regular exercise (5). A helpful guide on how to safely begin resistance training can be found, for example, in chapters five and six of the ACSM Fitness Book (6), which has very useful illustrations for beginners. A helpful guide for safety over the range of weightlifting workouts can be found in another ACSM publication (7). The key to becoming successful either in low-level resistance training or in weightlifting *per se* is to get instruction in proper technique at the beginning of your endeavors from a qualified trainer.

Although it is usually used for developing musculoskeletal fitness rather than cardiovascular fitness, weight training can be done aerobically, whether with machines or free weights. It all depends upon the routine you use. Neither power lifters nor body builders generally work out aerobically. Aiming for increased muscle strength and bulk, they are interested in lifting large amounts of weight for each "rep" (repetition) of the exercise in the "set" (the group of reps taken together), not necessarily in getting their heart rates up into the aerobic range. For them, the key is "high weight, low reps, low sets." They usually take a significant rest between each set, to allow the muscles time to recover. (In terms of number of participants, non-aerobic weightlifting is a major sport.)

However, lifting low weight with high reps in multiple sets, and taking little downtime between sets, can make the workout aerobic. At the same time, muscle flexibility and endurance will be increased. Some authorities recommend weight training as part of the exercise program for weight loss. In persons with a depressed resting metabolic rate, the only way to elevate it is to build up muscle mass, and of course weight training is a good way to do that.

You can lift weights at home or in a gym. If you plan on lifting free weights (barbells and dumbbells) at home without a partner, for safety reasons you should get instruction on the kinds of free-weight exercises you can do safely on your own (and there are many of them). In certain exercises, if while lifting you were to find yourself unable to support a given weight, you might get seriously injured putting it down, or worse, dropping it. Lifting on machines can be safely done on your own. But even with a home machine, before you start you should get some instruction in using it.

"Circuit training" is the name of an aerobic/resistance-training routine set up by some health clubs. A set of "stations" is assembled in a row or a circle. The progression through the circuit requires you to do an exercise at each station. In some cases the stations are arranged so that you will be alternating between aerobic and resistance exercises; some focus on resistance training alone. To give yourself a workout of the length that you need for that day, you can repeat the circuit as many times as you wish. Circuit training can be fun, especially because you are often doing it with other people on the circuit.

EQUIPMENT

Introduction

Choosing the right equipment and equipping yourself properly is as important as learning good technique, for many of the same reasons. Good equipment makes whatever sport or activity one is doing more comfortable, more fun. It also makes it safer in terms both of intrinsic (overuse and incorrect positional causes) and extrinsic (external causes) injury risk. As we have noted more than once, being comfortable while working out and avoiding injury both significantly increase the chances of sticking with regular exercise. It is not necessary to buy top-of-the-line, expensive equipment at the outset; good equipment, moderately priced, will do. As noted, most beginning scheduled leisure-time regular exercisers will start with walking, not an equipment-intensive sport. Later on, if one seriously gets into one of the "stuff" sports, there will be plenty of opportunity to spend money (as in lots of it). As far as clothing is concerned, at the beginning one will hopefully be able to find everything required, other than a good pair of shoes, right in the dresser and closet. Later on, once into it, the nice-looking stuff can be bought, possibly as a planned self-reward for exercise work well done. This book is not the place for a complete review of equipment requirements for all of the regular exercise sports. (For example, we do not cover treadmills, "elliptical machines," "steppers," rowing machines, and the like.) However, it provides enough information to get you started safely, at reasonable cost.

Shoes

For most of the sports that regular exercisers will engage in, the shoe is the single most important item of equipment. Not that the right shoe will convert an ordinary athlete into a superstar, as some shoe ads would have you believe. However, you will note that using the feet is central to the physical action of all of the sports we have covered other than swimming and weight training. Thus, when you make contact with the pavement, floor, machine platform, or pedal, the right foot-container can make the difference between feeling good and avoiding injury, and experiencing just the opposite.

There are several characteristics shared by good shoes for any sport. First, the shoe must fit well. Simply, the shoe should touch your foot in as many places as possible, except over the toes. For the toes, the "toe box" should be roomy, forward, laterally, and vertically. In other words, a good sport shoe should fit your foot like the right-size glove with no fingers fits your hand. Second, the shoe must be comfortable. While fitting snugly in the shoe, your foot should not be pinched, squeezed or squashed, causing pain at any point, whether you are standing still or moving. Third, for walking and running, people who "overpronate" (that is, when they land on each step they roll their ankle in too far, a common problem for many) should get shoes specifically designed to resist overpronation. If not compensated for, it is a common cause of injury further up the leg. A health fitness professional or a knowledgeable sport shoe salesperson will be able to tell you if you are an overpronator.

It is important that the shoe you use be specifically designed for the sport you choose. For example, PaceWalking™ shoes should be designed to give you cushioning, support, and to facilitate forward, not lateral, motion. Aerobic dance shoes should be designed to give you the flexibility and ease of lateral motion that you need for that sport. Correctly designed PaceWalking™ shoes will not work well for aerobic dance. By the same token, aerobic dance shoes will not be suitable for PaceWalking™. Cycling above the entry level requires special shoes of one sort or another.

Bicycles
PRINCIPAL CONSIDERATIONS

A great deal has been and can be written about bicycles and the many components and gadgets with which they can be equipped. Most of the brief comments offered here apply equally to road and mountain bikes. The most important design requirements for a bike are: it has a frame made of steel alloy (not straight non-alloy steel, even if it is described as "high tensile"; it is too heavy and too flexible), aluminum alloy, or some form of carbon fiber, it has aluminum alloy wheels. You want a bike that handles easily and is responsive (lightness), and one which transmits the power you are putting into the pedals into the rear, driving wheel, not into flexing the frame, thus wasting your effort (stiffness). Also, proper bike fit is very important. If the bike frame is either too large or too small for you, you will find it difficult and possibly painful and even dangerous to ride. You can get a decent road or mountain bicycle for $400.00 to $800.00 (2009 list prices). If you cannot afford to spend even the lower figure right now, wait. Unless it is on a special sale, a bike that costs much less than $400.00 (list) won't be worth buying.

OTHER BIKE EQUIPMENT

Right up there with the bike in importance is the hard-shell helmet. You should always wear a helmet when riding. A decent one will cost $50.00. You can spend more. Higher prices mean more comfort, more air vents, and cooler graphics, not more safety. (The helmet makers' insurance costs insure that they build as safe helmets as possible for any that they sell.) The cost of the helmet will be well worth it if you hit your head on the ground or pavement following a fall off your bike. To make sure that your helmet will stay on your head should you fall, make sure that the chin and ear straps are adjusted as tightly as comfort allows. Additional accessories include one-two water bottles, carried on the bike in "cages," a portable air pump and a spare tube and/or patch kit, and a small computer which can tell you your speed, distance, elapsed time, and in some cases cadence (pedal revolutions per minute). All of these accessories can be purchased for less than $200.00, including installation for those bits and pieces which need to be installed.

INDOOR BIKES

As far as indoor exercise bikes are concerned, you should look for: a well-built, rigid frame; a heavy, weighted flywheel that can give you the sensation of coasting just like a road bike, producing a smooth, not herky-jerky, ride; controls that are well-placed and easy-to-work; an easily adjustable, well-padded seat; legible instruments, if any; and toe-straps on the pedals so that, as with a road or mountain bike equipped with cleats, you can power the up-stroke as well as the down-stroke. You can get a very good indoor bicycle for $600–700.00 (and up, depending upon the computer/visual monitoring system included.) Obviously, you want to be sure that you would use such a device regularly and indefinitely before investing in one.

A more economical way to ride indoors is to mount a road bike on what is called an "indoor trainer." The important features of this device are that it clamps the bike firmly in place and provides a smooth, adjustable resistance. A good one costs $250–350.00. However, a road bike on a trainer does not provide as comfortable a ride as does an indoor exercise bike. One fun way to ride indoors is set your bike up in front of a television set or equip it with a reading stand. However, if you do either one, you have to remember to keep your cadence up or you won't get too much from the workout.

Weight-training Machines

Weightlifting can be done at home or in a gym. As noted above, for safety reasons, you have to limit the type of lifting with free weights (barbells and dumbbells) when done on your own. Wherever and with whomever you lift weights, you should do it only after receiving appropriate instruction. There are many types of home weight-training equipment, designed to provide for a variety of resistance exercises through a variety of cable-and-pulley arrangements and attachments. They can get to be quite expensive. It is important to note that regardless of cost, no machine or device can give you a "weightlifter's" body if you do not do a weightlifter's amount of work (which is way, way beyond the sometimes advertised "20 minutes/three times a week"). "Becoming muscular" requires lots of time, lots of work, and good training in the use of the equipment you are using, regardless of the kind of equipment you are using.

You can always incur intrinsic injury from trying to lift too much weight or lifting it the wrong way. However, since the resistance in a machine is provided either by a series of stacked weights or with bands or pistons that can be adjusted to provide a given resistance, it is highly unlikely that you could incur the type of crushing injuries that happen very occasionally with the use of free weights, used incorrectly and/or without a partner to "spot" you. Thus in most cases, you can generally use such machines safely alone.

Home resistance training weightlifting machines of various types range in price from under $100.00 to several thousand. At a minimum, you are looking at the $1000.00 range for a "multi-station gym" of good quality that you can safely use at home alone. The characteristics to look for are: main joints that are welded, not bolted (bolted main joints often being subject to working loose); any cables and pulleys should be made entirely of steel (aluminum cable and plastic pulleys wear easily); the quality of the rubber bands, springs, or hydraulic mechanisms used in some home machines is difficult to judge, but they should look neat and well-made; a well-padded bench; enough different stations so that you can get a full body workout, with variety; and it should be easy to make the seat position and any cable changes necessary for the different exercises.

As with any expensive piece of equipment, before purchasing a home weight-training machine you should be convinced that you are going to use it over the long term. If you are contemplating weightlifting for your regular exercise program, before buying a machine consider joining a health club known to have a good weight-training program and qualified instructors, at least for a trial membership. See if you like the sport. If you do, you may just decide to stick with the club. Or you can then go out and buy a good machine with confidence that you will make use of it.

CHOOSING A HEALTH CLUB

A health club or gym can be viewed as a collection of equipment that you rent for some time period, short or long, with staffing. You can use it either as a place where you try out various sports and routines which you plan eventually to do on your own, or as the place where you will be doing your program of regular exercise on an ongoing basis. In either case, it is useful to have a few guidelines that can help you choose a good one (6, p. 167–68). The club should be reasonably close to home or work, easy to get to, and, if you will be driving to it, have plenty of safe, adjacent parking. It should have convenient hours, open both early and late. Cleanliness in both the locker rooms and the workout areas is very important, both for your comfort and as an indication of how well the club and its equipment are managed and maintained. All areas should be well-lit for safety.

There should be ample staff. You should recognize that they have two jobs, helping members with their exercise routines is one. Selling new memberships as well as extensions and renewals is the other. You want to be certain that the pressure to undertake the latter function does not interfere with their ability and availability to carry out the former. For the former, staff should be both knowledgeable about regular exercise and the various sports and activities which you can do at the club, and be interested in helping you, especially at the beginning.

Ask about safety and the availability of staff trained in cardio-pulmonary resuscitation (CPR). Find out how many, if any, of the staff are certified in exercise supervision by one of the several certifying organizations, such as the American College of Sports Medicine, the Aerobics and Fitness Association of America, the International Dance-Exercise Association, or the Institute for Aerobics Research. If individual trainers are available, find out what their qualifications are. (Having an individual trainer is an extra cost item.)

The club should offer the sports/activities and machines/facilities in which you are interested. Virtually all will have free weights, at least one type of weight machine circuit, exercise bicycles, cross-country ski machines, stair climbers, steppers, "elliptical trainers," rowing machines, treadmills, and various kinds of aerobics classes. There should be enough equipment and classes to accommodate members without too much waiting at peak periods. Some clubs have an indoor track and/or a lap swimming pool, both very nice features.

Most clubs offer several different types of membership. When you visit a club, be sure to ask what "specials" are on. You may find especially attractive rates if your schedule permits you to make use of the club during off-peak hours. While most clubs are out to sign you up to a long-term contract, an increasing number are offering short-term trial and/or pay-by-the-month memberships. In general, it is cheaper to sign up for the long term than on a per-week or per-month basis. Nevertheless, as a rule-of-thumb, it is not a good idea to sign a long-term contract on your very first visit to the very first club you walk into. Check out several, make sure that you get their best deal, and make sure that you have dealt with the "regular" part of regular exercise first, so that any investment you make up front won't go to waste.

CLOTHING

Now that you have decided what exercise/sport(s) you are going to do, where you are going to do it, and with what equipment, we come to the clothing you can do it in. You can spend a lot of money on regular exercise and aerobic sports clothing. But you need not do so. If you cannot assemble a basic wardrobe for your sport or sports of choice from your closet and dresser, you can do so for any one sport for under $100.00.

As a general rule, clothing should be comfortable and loose-fitting. For all the sports requiring shoes, you should wear socks to help avoid blisters. A jogging bra is recommended for women. Under their shorts, men should wear support briefs or an athletic supporter. An increasing number of both men and women are finding that "compression shorts" (like bike shorts less the seat padding) are very comfortable for doing a wide variety of indoor and outdoor sports.

There are great, modern fabrics, bright colors, and flattering styles available in clothing for all of the aerobic sports. But when starting out, it is best to spend your money on the necessary equipment first. Then, when you are certain that you are going to stick with the sport, that you really like it, then you can spend money on that spiffy-looking, latest-style garment you saw down at the running shoe, cycling, or sporting goods store.

For cold-weather exercise outdoors, you should wear several layers of light-to-moderate weight garments rather than one heavier-weight set. Above all, you want clothing that is able to "breathe," that is let out through the fabric the moisture that accumulates as you get warm and sweat. On a chilly day, when starting out, you should wear just enough clothing to feel just a little on the chilly side yourself. If you feel nice and toasty warm at the beginning of a workout on a cold day, you are sure to feel hot and uncomfortable well before you finish it. No matter how cold it is, once you get going for a bit, you will begin to perspire.

CHRONOMETER

You will need a chronometer (digital stopwatch), to time your workouts, to check your heart rate, and, if you are biking and don't have a computer, to count your cadence. At a mass-market retailer, you can buy a decent digital watch for as little as $10.00, depending on its characteristics. Most important is that you should not be required to have a degree in mechanical engineering to set the device. You do not need a watch that is waterproof down to a depth of 300 meters below the water's surface. You are hardly likely to be doing your TSTEP down there. But a modicum of waterproofing is nice, say to 50 ft. Then you don't have to worry should you get caught out, or purposely go out, in the rain, and you can use it when you go swimming. A heart rate monitor, either combined with a chronometer or as a separate piece of equipment, is very helpful in keeping track of the intensity of your workouts (8).

CHOOSING A STORE

Your choice of store is very important in buying equipment of any type, whether it be shoes or bikes or weight-training machines or indoor rowers. Generally, do not buy regular exercise and sports equipment in department stores. In helping you select the equipment that is right for you, knowledgeable salespeople are critically important. Rarely will you find knowledgeable salespeople in department stores. While general sporting goods stores, the kind that outfits the local high school football team, may have knowledgeable salespeople when it comes to, say, shoes, that is not necessarily the case. The quality of the "stuff" and the staff in sporting goods "superstores" varies widely. If they come across as knowledgeable, that's fine. However, as a general rule, it is a good idea to patronize specialty shops.

It is a good idea, for example, to buy at least your first pair of PaceWalking™, running, or indoor aerobic exercise shoes from a store that specializes in athletic shoes. You will decide, of course what looks and feels good to you. But it is the salesperson in the running shoe store, dealing with the product every day, who is most likely to be able to give you proper advice on the characteristics of the various shoes that the store carries and proper fit. Most such stores are staffed by people who are athletes themselves, can speak to you from personal experience, and can intelligently interpret for you the comments of other users of a particular shoe.

As for bikes, buy only in a bike store. You will be best off in what is called a "pro shop," one staffed with riders and patronized by people who wear hardshell helmets and black bike shoes. The most expensive bike in the store should sell for at least twice what you are planning to spend. If it does, you know that you are in a store where the staff most likely knows what it is doing. They have to. The same advice goes for buying weight/resistance-training equipment: buy it in a shop that has knowledgeable sales people. In any kind of aerobic sports equipment store, if you feel that the person really doesn't know what they are talking about, ask to see the manager. If none is available to talk with you, go somewhere else.

CONCLUSION

Both technique and equipment are meant to serve you, not the other way round. Unless you intend to become a higher-end participant/competitor in the sport(s) you have chosen, once you have learned the basics of technique, focus on becoming and staying regular with it/them and having fun at the same time (see Chapter 15). As we said at the outset of this chapter, becoming a technique fanatic when you don't need to be is one sure way to take the enjoyment out of your exercising and lead you straight to quitting. Likewise, one can become an equipment fanatic. Too many indoor exercise machines of various kinds end up being clothes drying racks and too many fancy bikes just hang in the garage from year to year. Before you make any major investments in exercise equipment, be sure that you have dealt with the hard part of regular exercise, that is, the regular, first. Once you are a *regular* exerciser, there will be plenty of time to acquire suitable and even fancy equipment. If you use it regularly, then you will be able to really enjoy it.

References

1. Sheehan G. Running wild. *Phys Sports Med.* 1986 Oct.
2. Lobb W. Founding father of fitness. *Runner's World.* 1993 June, 1993, p. 16.
3. Jonas S., Radetsky P. *PaceWalking: the balanced way to aerobic health.* New York: Crown; 1988. 215 p.
4. Jonas S. Regular exercise: a handbook for clinical practice. New York: Springer Publishing Co.; 1995. 238 p.
5. ACSM: "Physical Activity & Public Health Guidelines" (with the American Heart Association), 2008, at www.acsm.org.
6. American College of Sports Medicine (US). *ACSM fitness book.* 3rd ed. Champaign (IL): Human Kinetics; c2003. Chapter 5, Beginning exercises; p. 89–120. Chapter 6, The ACSM Fitness Program; p. 121–152.
7. Bird M. Building strength safely. [Internet] ACSM *Fit Society Page.* 2002; Fall:3. [cited 2008 Sep 28]. Available from: http://www.acsm.org/AM/Template.cfm?Section=Search&TEMPLATE=/CM/ContentDisplay.cfm&CONTENTID=1273
8. See, for example, Heart Zones USA [Internet]. Sacramento (CA): Heart Zones USA; c2008 [cited 2008 Sep 28]. Available from: http://www.heartzones.com

CHAPTER 13

Special Conditions

Edward M. Phillips

INTRODUCTION

Much of the material covered thus far addresses exercise prescription and the benefits of physical activity in the apparently healthy patient. Many of your patients, however, will present with illnesses or conditions that will impact their ability to undertake and continue a program of physical activity. In Chapter 3, we covered screening of these individuals to best assure their safety in initiating, maintaining, or increasing physical activity. In this chapter, we will focus on 10 different prevalent conditions and detail the use of exercise in managing these conditions or performing exercise with the conditions.

Despite the diversity of the conditions detailed in this chapter, the exercise prescription often follows the general recommendations for apparently healthy adults. In each section, we will focus on modifications and precautions to this general recommendation (Figure 13.1).

For each condition we will follow roughly the same format to make it easier for you to quickly find the salient information:

- Illness or Condition
- Definition
- Prevalence and Incidence
- Other treatments (medication, surgery, etc.)
- Testing and screening, with reference to Chapter 3
- Precautions
- Exercise Prescription: Modifications from general recommendations

This selection of illnesses and conditions is not meant to be exhaustive. A more thorough description of the use of exercise in 46 conditions may be found in ACSM's Exercise Management for Persons with Chronic Disease and Disability Book (1) or in the Guidelines for Exercise Prescription and Testing, Chapter 10, on Special Conditions (2). The following represent prevalent conditions that your patient will likely present:

- Arthritis
- Hypertension

SPAULDING REHABILITATION HOSPITAL
125 NASHUA STREET
BOSTON, MASSACHUSETTS 02114
617-573-7000

SPAULDING
REHABILITATION
HOSPITAL
N E T W O R K

PATIENT'S FULL NAME	PHONE NUMBER	AGE	SEX

ADDRESS	DATE / /

℞ Moderate intensity physical activity, 30 minutes per day, at least 5 days per week but preferably all days of the week, or vigorous intensity exercise 20 minutes three days per week or combination. May accumulate in bouts of at least 10 minutes.
Avoid two consecutive days of inactivity.
Resistance exercise 2 days per week; one-three sets of eight-12 repetitions to point of fatigue with last repetition.

☐ Refills   1   2   3   4   (Forever)
☐ No Refills   Void After _____

DEA: _____

Dr: *Edward Phillips, M.D.*

Interchange mandated unless the practitioner writes the words "No Subsitution" in this space

VALID FOR CONTROLLED SUBSTANCES

Figure 13.1 • Exercise Prescription for Healthy Adult.

- Overweight/Obesity
- Osteoporosis
- Pregnancy
- Cancer
- Cardiovascular Disease
- Older Adults
- Depression
- Diabetes

ARTHRITIS

Definition

While there are over 100 rheumatic diseases, the most common conditions that your patients will present with include osteoarthritis and rheumatoid arthritis (3, 4). Osteoarthritis, or degenerative joint disease, primarily affects the joints in the weight bearing regions of the spine, hips, and knees, but often affects the hands as well. Rheumatoid arthritis is a condition of pathological activity of the immune system that commonly affects the joints.

Incidence and Prevalence

By 2020 more than 60 million people in the United States will be affected by these conditions. More than 80% of your patients above the age of 65 will present with some evidence of degenerative joint disease (osteoarthritis).

Other Treatments (5)

- Weight loss
- Education in self-management
- Patient support groups
- Appropriate footwear to reduce shock to lower extremities
- Occupational Therapy
- Physical Therapy
- Assistive devices (canes, walkers, bracing)
- Non-steroidal anti-inflammatory medications
- Disease modifying medications for rheumatoid arthritis
- Surgery for joint debridement and total joint replacement

Benefits of Exercise

- Strengthening and maintenance of muscle strength around joints from resistance training
- Reduced joint stiffness from stretching and physical activity

Screening

Avoid vigorous-intensity physical activity if there is an acutely inflamed joint being exercised. If lower extremity arthritis prevents comfortably walking on a treadmill or using a bicycle, consider using upper extremity exercise with an arm ergometer (a bicycle device for the arms). Be especially careful to allow for adequate warm-up time at a low intensity before pursuing a more strenuous exercise test. Isotonic, isokinetic, or isometric muscle strength can be assessed (2).

Exercise Prescription

As with many other conditions, the general recommendation for FITT (Frequency, Intensity, Time, and Type) follows those for apparently healthy adults.

Modifications: Your patients with acutely or chronically painful knees and hips commonly complain that even walking is difficult. You may recommend exercises with low stress across the lower extremity joints including bicycling, swimming, or walking in the water to reduce the effects of gravity. Exercise in warm water 83°–88°F (28–31°C) helps with pain reduction and relaxation of the muscles. Walking may be aided by a cane to partially unweight joints. As your patient progresses, emphasize increasing the time rather than the intensity of their activity.

Resistance training will directly strengthen the muscle weakness around the affected joint. This may comfortably begin with isometric contractions, such as straight leg raises for a painful knee that do not involve moving the affected joint. As your patient becomes stronger and more comfortable, you may then advise him to progress to isotonic training of the affected joints.

Stretching helps maintain flexibility. Gentle movement through the full available range of motion may safely be advised even when your patient experiences inflammation and pain.

Patient Education

Patients should understand the vital role of resistance training to help maintain strong muscles around the affected joint, and will reduce stress across the joint. For example, strengthening the quadriceps and hamstrings will provide support to arthritic knees. Arthritic patients who initiate a program of exercise must understand that some discomfort while exercising or for two hours after they exercise should be expected, and does not indicate that they are injuring their joints. If the pain continues well after the first two hours or exceeds their general level of joint pain, they should be counseled to reduce the duration and/or intensity in their next session. It is quite reasonable to time the exercises with their period of least severity of pain and/or after taking pain medications.

The impact of arthritic conditions on your patient's function is critical. As such, exercises may appropriately focus on maintaining common activities such as transferring from sit-to-stand or step-ups to maintain independence in daily living.

HYPERTENSION

Definition

Hypertension is defined by a resting systolic blood pressure (SBP) ≥140 mm Hg and/or diastolic blood pressure (DBP) ≥ 90 mm Hg. Blood pressure as low as 120/80 mm Hg is considered pre-hypertension (6) and puts your patient at a higher risk for ischemic heart disease and stroke. See Table 13.1 for blood pressure classification scheme. Essential hypertension, where the cause of the high blood pressure is not known, accounts for 90% of the incidence.

Incidence and Prevalence

Approximately 65 million Americans have high blood pressure. A majority of your older patients will have hypertension. Fortunately, the beneficial reduction of blood pressure through exercise occurs regardless of age.

TABLE 13.1 Classification and Management of Blood Pressure for Adults†

BP Classification	SBP mm Hg	DBP mm Hg	Lifestyle Modification	Initial Drug Therapy	
				Without Compelling Indication	With Compelling Indications
Normal	<120	And <80	Encourage	No	
Prehypertension	120–139	Or 80–89	Yes	No antihypertensive drug indicated	Drug(s) for compelling indications.‡
Stage 1 Hypertension	140–159	Or 90–99	Yes	Antihypertensive drug(s) indicated	Drug(s) for compelling indications.‡ Other antihypertensive drugs, as needed.
Stage 2 Hypertension	≥160	Or ≥100	Yes	Antihypertensive drug(s) indicated. Two-drug combination for most.§	

†Treatment determined by highest BP category.

‡Compelling indications include heart failure, post-myocardial infarction, high coronary heart disease risk, diabetes, chronic kidney disease, and recurrent stroke prevention. Treat patients with chronic kidney disease or diabetes to BP goal of <130/80 mm Hg.

§Initial combined therapy should be used cautiously in those at risk for orthostatic hypotension.

Abbreviations: DBP, diastolic blood pressure; SBP, systolic blood pressure.

Adapted from National High Blood Pressure Education Program. The seventh report of the Joint National Committee on Prevention, Detection, Evaluation, and Treatment of High Blood Pressure (JNC7). 2003; 3:5233.

Other Treatments
- Weight loss
- DASH Diet (Dietary Approaches to Stop Hypertension)
- Medications

Benefits of Exercise

Reductions of 5–7 mm Hg are achieved in patients who are hypertensive who maintain an aerobic training program (7). Blood pressure is also lowered at submaximal exercise workloads. Immediately after aerobic exercise, your patient will experience lower blood pressure from post-exercise hypotension.

Because of the marked overlap of overweight/obesity and hypertension, the exercise program should be designed to help with weight reduction and maintenance of weight loss. This will involve working toward a longer period of exercise each week. (Please see Overweight/Obesity section below.)

Screening

Patients with resting SBP ≥ 200 mm Hg or DBP ≥ 110 mm Hg should not undergo exercise testing nor be allowed to exercise. Patients on beta-blockers may have reduced exercise capacity during testing due to the medication. Because of the chronotropic effect of these medications, the patient's perceived exertion might be a more appropriate measure than heart rate during screening and exercise sessions.

Exercise Prescription

As with many other conditions, the general recommendation for FITT (Frequency, Intensity, Time, and Type) follows those for apparently healthy adults with the following precautions.

Your patients are stratified into three different risk groups according to their blood pressure level and presence of other cardiovascular risk factors, target organ damage, or clinical cardiovascular disease (see Table 13.1 Blood Pressure Classification). While patients with hypertension need medical evaluation before formal exercise testing, the majority of your patients with hypertension can safely initiate moderate-intensity aerobic exercise. If the patient is in the most-severe risk group and wishes to pursue moderate-intensity exercise, he should be referred for a symptom-limited graded exercise test. The same recommendation holds for any hypertensive patient who would like to train at a vigorous intensity.

During resistance training, your patient should be instructed to avoid Valsalva maneuver by learning to breathe throughout the exercise. If your patient is being treated with alpha-blocker, calcium channel blocker, or vasodilators, she must be instructed to watch for sudden reductions in blood pressure after exercise. These patients should be monitored during exercise and in the cool-down period. Diuretic therapy may induce hypokalemia or cardiac dysrhythmias. Diuretics and beta-blockers may cause hypoglycemia in some individuals (see Diabetes section, below). These same medications may affect thermoregulatory function and cause heat intolerance. Exercise capacity may be reduced by beta-blockers. Exercise should be stopped for SBP ≥250 mm Hg and/or DBP ≥115 mm Hg.

Patients with cardiovascular disease (ischemic heart disease, heart failure, or stroke) may undergo vigorous-intensity exercise training under medical supervision.

OVERWEIGHT AND OBESITY

Definition, Prevalence, and Incidence

More than 66% of American adults are classified as overweight as indicated by a BMI ≥25 kg/m². Nearly one-third are obese, with BMI ≥30 kg/m², and 5% are extremely obese, with BMI ≥40 kg/m² (8). As a rule of thumb, if your 5-foot-3-inch female patient is 30 pounds overweight, she is considered obese. As detailed in Chapter 14, obesity is a rising concern for children and adolescents with 14%–18% overweight. In youth, overweight is classified as ≥85th percentile of BMI for age and gender (8).

Other Treatments

- Medications
- Bariatric surgery
- Weight loss regimens through caloric restriction
- Support groups

Weight management boils down to finding the proper balance of energy intake and energy expenditure. For your patients who have habitually taken in more calories than they use, the result is an excess of energy stored as fat. Rebalancing so that your patient expends more than he takes in will result in weight loss. An appropriate weight loss goal for overweight and obese individuals to achieve significant health benefits (9) is 5%–10%. This rather modest weight loss goal (as little as a 15-pound loss in a 300-pound individual) is consistent with the discussion in the chapters on motivation (Chapters 4–6) that stress setting achievable goals and taking small steps to begin the process. Even so, maintaining weight loss is notoriously difficult, with one-third to half of weight regained within a year of completing the diet or medication regimen (10).

Weight loss regimens with reduced caloric intake and increased burning of calories through more physical activity and exercise result in 9%–10% loss of weight (10). Interestingly, physical activity has little impact on the amount of weight lost in the first six months, compared to dieting (9); however, adequate physical activity is critical to maintaining weight loss (11). Stated another way, exercise alone won't get the weight off, but exercise is essential to keeping the weight off.

Meeting the recommended minimal physical activity with moderate-intensity exercise at around 6 calories per minute performed for at least 150 minutes per week results in approximately 900 kcal of energy expenditure in exercise. The National Weight Control Registry at the University of Colorado reports that individuals who have lost at least 30 kilograms and kept this weight off for at least five years maintain weekly exercise of 2800 kcal (12).

Testing and Screening

The co-morbidities commonly associated with overweight and obesity (*e.g.,* hypertension, diabetes, and heart disease) may increase the required level of screening before exercise testing or commencing an exercise regimen. With obese individuals, walking on a treadmill may not be practical. Testing or exercise on a cycle with an appropriate seat may be appropriate. Anticipate extremely low exercise capacity in patients who are overweight and obese. Start exercise as low as 2–3 METs and advance as slowly as 0.5 METs during testing or exercise sessions.

Exercise Prescription: Modifications From General Recommendations

For overweight and obese patients, the general recommendations for the exercise prescription follow those of apparently healthy adults for aerobics, resistance, and flexibility. The minimum dose of 150 minutes per week of moderately intense physical activity confers the general health benefits. The modification for overweight and obese patients is to increase the frequency to five or more days per week to maximize caloric expenditure. Intensity may start at moderate and increase to vigorous to obtain higher levels of physical fitness. Similarly, time in exercise should be increased from 30 minutes to 60 minutes daily (or longer), again to burn more calories. The type of exercise will generally involve large muscle groups, such as walking or cycling. Resistance training will help balance the exercise program.

OSTEOPOROSIS

Definition

Osteoporosis is a disease of the bones characterized by low bone mineral density (BMD) and susceptibility to fracture from alteration of the microarchitecture of the bone. Osteoporosis in postmenopausal women and men 50 years of age or older is defined by BMD T-score of the lumbar spine, total hip, or femoral neck of more than 2.5 standard deviations below the young adult mean value, with or without accompanying fractures (13–16). Your patients are at risk for fractures even if their BMD scores are above this threshold, especially if the patients are elderly. Hip fractures are associated with the greatest increased risk of death and disability.

Incidence and Prevalence

More than 10 million Americans 50 years of age and older have osteoporosis and another 34 million are at risk (17).

Benefits of Exercise

- Decreased osteoporotic fractures by increased peak bone mass
- Slowed rate of bone loss with aging
- Reduced fall risk due to improved muscle strength and balance (18, 19)
- Higher bone mass achieved in childhood, adolescence, and young adulthood through adequate physical activity is maintained into adulthood

Other Treatments

- Dietary or supplementation of calcium
- Vitamin D supplementation and/or exposure to sunlight
- Hormone Replacement: Estrogen and progesterone
- Medications

Precautions

"There are currently no established guidelines regarding contraindications for exercise for people with osteoporosis" (2). Common sense prevails, however, and patients should be advised to stay away from any exercise that causes or exacerbates pain. Twisting, bending, or compression of the spine and high impact loading or explosive movements should be avoided. As such, maximal muscle strength testing may be contraindicated in patients with severe osteoporosis. Forward flexion of the spine, even without loading, places the spine at greatly increased risk of spinal compression fractures (20).

If your patient has severe vertebral osteoporosis, then alternatives to walking may be preferable when choosing the type of exercise.

Balance may be affected by the forward shift in the center of gravity in patients with vertebral compression fractures. As discussed in exercise for older adults, exercises to improve balance and reduce the chances of falling should be addressed. Even the frailest older adults should be prescribed an activity regimen to avoid further bone loss from bed rest.

Exercise Prescription

To preserve bone health, prescribe exercise in your patients *at risk* for osteoporosis as defined by low bone mass, age, and female gender (17).

Frequency: *Weight-bearing* aerobic activities three to five days per week, and resistance exercise two to three days per week

Intensity: Moderate (eight to 12 repetitions for resistance exercise) to high intensity (five to six repetitions for resistance exercise); moderate-intensity aerobic activity (40–60% of HRR) (see Chapter 8 for definitions.)

Time: 30 to 60 minutes per day, combination of weight bearing aerobic and resistance activities

Type: Weight-bearing aerobic activities include walking and intermittent jogging, stair climbing, or tennis. Your patients may also pursue exercises that involve jumping, such as volleyball and basketball. These types of exercise help to stimulate strengthening of the bones. In addition, back-strengthening exercises (while avoiding flexion of the spine) can help the supporting muscles of the spine and thereby reduce spine fractures (20).

For patients *with* osteoporosis, the previous exercise prescription may be modified to avoid the high-intensity resistance exercises, although patients may be able to progress to this level. Patients with osteoporosis will not be encouraged to pursue jumping exercises or running. Non-weight-bearing exercises, such as swimming and bicycling, still confer general health benefits, muscle strengthening, and some improvements in bone health through muscle traction on the bone.

PREGNANCY

Definition

Unlike most of the conditions covered in this chapter, pregnancy is not a disease or illness. Like many other medical conditions, however, pregnancy does cause physiological changes in the body that can influence exercise participation and potentially make clinicians wary of prescribing exercise. The American College of Obstetrics and Gynecology (ACOG) and the ACSM recommend that exercise is just as important during pregnancy. Despite these recommendations, studies have shown that pregnant women (excluding those whose pregnancies are considered high-risk) are less likely to be meeting the ACSM/AHA-recommended exercise levels (21). Therefore, as a clinician, it is particularly important to recommend exercise to patients who are currently or planning to become pregnant, with the exception of women whose pregnancies are classified as high-risk (see high-risk pregnancy below). As well as the general benefits of exercise, pregnant women are encouraged to exercise so as to have less fatigue, to benefit from better control of weight gain, and to possibly experience shorter labor (22).

Pregnancy causes a number of physiological changes in the body's response to exercise. Although it is important to appreciate these changes, they should not prohibit most women from participating in an exercise program while pregnant. With respect to its effect on exercise, one of the most significant changes is the increase in resting energy expenditure resulting in increased effort required to exercise (23). This increased energy consumption results in a higher $\dot{V}O2$ (oxygen consumption), cardiac output, and stroke volumes; however, maximal heart rate appears to remain unchanged (23). Increases in energy expenditure also result in a greater difficulty removing heat from the body. Table 13.2 provides some tips to help pregnant women avoid overheating while exercising.

Benefits

- Maintenance of prenatal aerobic and musculoskeletal fitness levels
- Prevention of excessive maternal weight gain
- Facilitation of labor and recovery from labor
- Promotion of good posture
- Prevention of gestational glucose intolerance
- Prevention of low back pain
- Improved psychological adjustment to the changes of pregnancy (24, 25)

Exercise Screening and Testing

Clearly, women who are pregnant are not immune to other medical conditions such as diabetes or cardiovascular disease. Therefore, the medical screening described in Chapter 3 should still be applied to pregnant women who want to begin an exercise program. Gestational diabetes mellitus is one of the most common complications of pregnancy (26, 27). In addition to the general medical screening described in Chapter 3, the ACOG recommends using the "Physical Activity Readiness Medical Examination for Pregnancy," published

---

TABLE 13.2 Exercise Tips for Pregnant Women

- Changes in body shape and weight will affect balance. Avoid unstable positions and take extra care not to fall
- Drink plenty of fluids before, during, and after exercising
- Avoid overheating while exercising:
  - Dress in layers and wear comfortable, loose-fitting clothes that permit evaporation of sweat
  - Exercise in cooler or well-ventilated places (or times of the day)
  - Avoid swimming in warm or hot water and avoid immersion in hot tubs
  - Be aware of the early symptoms of heat illness: nausea, dizziness, headache, poor coordination, and apathy.
- Set realistic exercise goals, bearing in mind the fact that exercise will become more difficult as the pregnancy progresses
- Avoid exercising on your back (supine) in the second and third trimesters

Adapted from: Soultanakis-aligianni, 2003, and Thompson, 2007

by the same group as the PAR-Q (see Chapter 3) (22). This easy-to-use screening tool is freely available at http://www.csep.ca/forms.asp.

Exercise Prescription

The American College of Obstetrics and Gynecology (ACOG) recommends that pregnant women should exercise with similar safeguards as non-pregnant women, provided that there are no medical or obstetric complications during the pregnancy (22, 28, 29). Most women who were active before pregnancy can and should continue to exercise (22, 28). Early in the pregnancy, previously active women may continue to train at their prepregnancy parameters (frequency, time/duration, intensity, and type). These parameters should naturally decrease and be modified, as the pregnancy progresses (22). In general, women who were sedentary prior to their pregnancy and whose pregnancies are not considered high-risk are safe to begin a low- or moderate-intensity program (22).

Based on these recommendations (28), the following exercise prescription is recommended for pregnant women without medical or obstetric complications:

Frequency: Same as ACSM/AHA recommendations: at least five times per week if exercising at moderate intensity, and at least three times each week if exercising at vigorous intensity

Intensity: For women who were previously sedentary, begin exercising at low to moderate intensity. Women who were previously active are initially encouraged to continue exercise at the same intensity (30). As the pregnancy progresses, the intensity usually decreases naturally (22).

Time: Same as ACSM/AHA recommendations

Type: The type of exercise that pregnant women participate in is a matter of personal choice. Contact sports, scuba diving, or other activities that might possibly cause abdominal distress should be avoided during pregnancy (30). In addition, exercise performed in a supine position is not recommended after the first trimester, because the weight of the fetus on the vena cava restricts venous return and cardiac output (23).

Many women who were active prior to becoming pregnant will choose to continue with their chosen sports (and routine). For those women just beginning a program, again the choice is theirs; however, the following information may influence their choices. Walking is the most popular choice of exercise for pregnant (and non pregnant) women (21); however, the energy expended during weight-supported exercises (such as walking) increases during pregnancy. This increased energy expenditure is primarily due to increased body weight (23). Therefore, non-weight-supported exercises (*e.g.,* cycling or swimming) may be preferable for pregnant women. Water activities (such as water aerobics or swimming) are an ideal environment for pregnant women to exercise in (providing the water is not too hot) (31, 32). In addition to being non-weight-bearing and providing buoyancy to counter the additional weight of the growing fetus, exercising in water may facilitate venous return as a result of the water's external hydrostatic pressure (23).

Due to the stretching and potential injury to the muscles of the pelvic floor during labor and delivery, as well as the additional weight of the fetus on the pelvic floor, exercises to strengthen the pelvic floor are recommended both during pregnancy and postpartum (although additional randomized control studies are needed to assess the long-term benefits) (33). These exercises, sometimes referred to as "Kegel exercises," are the first line of treatment for urinary incontinence (33).

Special Considerations and Precautions
HIGH-RISK PREGNANCY

In general, women who have high-risk pregnancies should avoid exercise. This includes women with pregnancy-induced hypertension, poorly controlled type 1 diabetes, and women experiencing persistent second- or third-trimester bleeding (22). Table 13.3 lists both absolute and relative contraindications to

---

TABLE 13.3 Contraindications to Exercise during Pregnancy

Absolute contraindications to exercise during pregnancy (ACOG)

- History of three or more spontaneous miscarriages
- Ruptured membranes
- Premature labor
- Diagnosed multiple pregnancies, *e.g.,* twins, triplets
- Intrauterine growth retardation (baby is smaller than expected)
- Incompetent cervix (cervix becomes softer and more open than normal)
- Placenta previa (portion of the placenta sits over the cervix, making it more vulnerable to detachment)
- Pregnancy-induced hypertension
- Venous thrombosis or pulmonary embolism (clots to legs or lungs)
- Known cardiac valve disease
- Primary pulmonary hypertension
- Maternal heart disease

Relative contraindications to exercise (medical clearance required) (ACOG)

- Hypertension
- Anemia
- Thyroid disease
- Diabetes
- Extremely over- or underweight
- Extremely sedentary
- Breech presentation in third trimester
- History of bleeding during pregnancy

exercise. Further, as per the recommendations in Chapter 3, women with cardiovascular, pulmonary, or metabolic disease should undergo further medical testing and should be monitored by a physician if they are able to exercise during pregnancy (22).

GESTATIONAL DIABETES MELLITUS (GDM)

Most women who develop gestational diabetes mellitus (GDM) will still benefit from regular physical activity (at low or moderate intensity). According to the American Diabetes Association (34), "regular physical activity can help lower fasting and postprandial plasma glucose concentrations and may be used as an adjunct to improve maternal glycemia." In addition, exercise can help to control excessive gestational weight gain (27), a relatively common complication of diabetes.

CANCER

Definition

Cancer is characterized by uncontrolled growth and spread of abnormal cells from damage to DNA by internal factors (*e.g.,* inherited mutations) and/or environmental exposure (*e.g.,* tobacco smoke) (2). Cancer arises from different cell types and has a lifetime prevalence of one out of two in men and one out of three in women (35). More than three-quarters of cancers are diagnosed in patients 55 years and older (35).

Other Treatments

- Surgery
- Radiation
- Chemotherapy
- Hormones
- Immunotherapy

Due to the cancer as well as to the side effects of some treatments damaging healthy tissues, patients often report limitations in their exercise capacity during and after treatment. Even five years and more after treatment, more than half of cancer patients report significant physical performance restrictions for standing, walking, and lifting (36).

Screening

Cancer and cancer therapy can affect multiple components of physical fitness, including cardiovascular capacity, muscular strength and endurance, body composition, flexibility, gait, and balance (2). As such, clinicians need to complete a comprehensive evaluation to address the cancer, the side effects of the treatment, and the common co-morbidities, including cardiopulmonary disease, diabetes mellitus, osteoporosis, and arthritis, which are all common in older adults.

A medically supervised symptom-limited or maximal exercise test is strongly recommended in cancer patients initiating an exercise regimen. Alternatively, a submaximal exercise test can assess the patient at least to the anticipated level of the planned daily exercise.

Exercise Prescription

There are no firm guidelines for precise recommendations of the exercise prescription in patients with cancer. The American Cancer Society supports the use of the exercise prescription for otherwise healthy individuals.

Frequency: Aerobics three to five days per week. Resistance exercise two to three days per week (with at least 48 hours between sessions). Flexibility exercise two to seven days per week. Table 13.4 lists the contraindications and precautions to exercise testing and training in patients with cancer.

CARDIOVASCULAR DISEASE

Benefits of Exercise

The extensive screening and referral process for patients with cardiovascular disease should not be misconstrued as a suggestion that exercise is not beneficial or recommended for patients with cardiovascular disease (or its risk factors). The American Heart Association strongly emphasizes that exercise is a valuable therapeutic strategy for patients with, or at risk for, atherosclerotic cardiovascular disease (37).

In 2003, the American Heart Association issued a statement, endorsed by the American College of Sports Medicine, on physical activity and atherosclerotic cardiovascular disease: "regular physical activity using large muscle groups, such as walking, running, or swimming, produces cardiovascular adaptations that increase exercise capacity, endurance, and skeletal muscle strength. Habitual physical activity also prevents the development of coronary artery disease (CAD) and reduces symptoms in patients with established cardiovascular disease" (38).

They state further that regular exercise can aid in the prevention of cardiovascular disease, as well as a number of atherosclerotic risk factors (38) (Table 13.5). Therefore, although careful screening of patients with cardiovascular disease or risk factors is necessary, encouraging patients with such conditions to develop an active lifestyle is vital. Depending on the severity of your patient's symptoms or risk factors, certain modifications may need to be made to her exercise program. In addition to the compelling evidence that exercise can play an important preventative role, the AHA statement also pro-

TABLE 13.4 Contraindications and Precautions to Exercise Testing and Training for Patients with Cancer

	Contraindications to exercise testing and training	Precautions requiring modification and/or physician approval
Factors related to cancer treatment	• No exercise on days of intravenous chemotherapy or within 24 h of treatment • No exercise prior to blood draw • Severe tissue reaction to radiation therapy	• Caution if on treatments that affect the lungs and/or heart: recommend medically supervised exercise testing and training • Mouth sores/ulcerations: avoid mouthpieces for maximal testing; use face masks
Hematologic	• Platelets <50,000 • White blood cells <3,000 • Hemoglobin <10 $g{\cdot}dL^{-1}$	• Platelets >50,000–150,000: avoid tests that increase risk of bleeding • White blood cells >3,000–4,000: ensure proper sterilization of equipment • Hemoglobin >10 $g{\cdot}dL^{-1}$ –11.5/13.5 $g{\cdot}dL^{-1}$: caution with maximal tests
Musculoskeletal	• Bone, back, or neck pain of recent origin • Unusual muscular weakness • Severe cachexia • Unusual/extreme fatigue • Poor functional status: avoid exercise testing if Karnofsky Performance Status score ≤60%	• Any pain or cramping: investigate • Osteopenia: avoid high-impact exercise if risk of fracture • Steroid induced myopathy • Cachexia: multidisciplinary approach to exercise • Mild to moderate fatigue: closely monitor response to exercise
Systemic	• Acute infections • Febrile illness: fever >100°F (38°C) • General malaise	• Recent systemic illness or infection: avoid exercise until asymptomatic for >48 h

TABLE 13.4 *(Continued)*

	Contraindications to exercise testing and training	Precautions requiring modification and/or physician approval
Gastrointestinal	• Severe nausea • Vomiting or diarrhea within 24–36 h • Dehydration • Poor nutrition: inadequate fluid and/or intake	• Compromised fluid and/or food intake: recommend multidisciplinary approach/consultation with nutritionist
Cardiovascular	• Chest pain • Resting HR >100 beats·min^{-1} or <50 beats·min^{-1} • Resting SBP >145 mm Hg and/or DBP >95 mm Hg • Resting SBP <85 mm Hg • Irregular HR • Swelling of ankles	• Caution if at risk of cardiac disease: recommend medically supervised exercise testing and training • If on antihypertensive medications that affect HR, THR may not be attainable; avoid overexertion • Lymphedema: wear compression garment on limb when exercising Mild to moderate dyspnea: avoid maximal tests
Pulmonary	• Severe dyspnea • Cough, wheezing • Chest pain increased by deep breath	• Mild cognitive changes: ensure that patient is able to understand and follow instructions
Neurologic	• Significant decline in cognitive status • Dizziness/lightheadedness • Disorientation • Blurred vision • Ataxia (i.e., inability to co-ordinate voluntary movement)	• Poor balance/peripheral sensory neuropathy: use well-supported positions for exercise

HR = heart rate; THR = target heart rate; SBP = systolic blood pressure.
Reprinted with permission from McNeely ML, Peddle C, Parliament M, Courneya KS. Cancer rehabilitation: recommendations for integrating exercise programming in the clinical practice setting. Curr Cancer Ther Rev. 2006 Nov;2(4):351–60.

TABLE 13.5 The Effect of Exercise on Atherosclerotic Risk Factors

- Decreases elevated blood pressure
- Lowers insulin resistance and glucose intolerance
- Lowers elevated triglyceride concentrations
- Lowers cholesterol (raises high-density lipoprotein cholesterol [HDL-C] concentrations, and, in combination with weight reduction, can decrease low-density lipoprotein cholesterol [LDL-C] concentrations)
- Prevents the onset of type 2 diabetes in individuals at high risk for this disease

Source: Thompson et al, 2003

vides strong recommendations for the use of exercise in the treatment of patients with cardiovascular diseases (38).

As we progress into a discussion of the cardiovascular risks associated with exercise and the treatment of patients with cardiovascular disease, we need to stress that clinicians working with patients at high risk for an acute cardiovascular event—such as during high-level exercise testing or inpatient treatment of patients following cardiac surgery—must have specific training in this area. This book is designed for patients in lower-risk categories, or those who have been safely discharged home following a cardiac event or surgery. For further information on the testing and treatment of high-risk cardiovascular patients, we refer you to the Guidelines for Exercise Testing and Prescription, 8th edition, Chapter 9, and the AHA Exercise Standards for Testing and Training: A Statement for Health Professionals from the American Heart Association (39).

Risk Stratification

In Chapter 3, we emphasized the importance of careful Risk Assessment and Exercise Screening of patients. One of the primary purposes of the assessment is to identify cardiovascular history, signs and symptoms, and risk factors. Those with a positive finding of cardiovascular disease, signs and symptoms, or numerous (≥2) risk factors are referred for further medical testing, or modifications of their exercise program are recommended.

The results of that testing and evaluation further stratify these patients into low-, moderate-, and high-risk groups (see Chapter 3). See Table 13.6 for the risk stratification of patients with known CVD.

Cardiovascular Risks Associated with Exercise

Vigorous physical activity has been shown to acutely increase the risk of sudden cardiac death and myocardial infarction among individuals with both diagnosed and occult cardiac conditions (38). Further, in adults, atheroscle-

TABLE 13.6 Risk Stratification

American Association of Cardiovascular and Pulmonary Rehabilitation Risk Stratification Criteria for Cardiac Patients

LOWEST RISK

Characteristics of patients at lowest risk for exercise participation (all characteristics listed must be present for patients to remain at lowest risk)

- Absence of complex ventricular dysrhythmias during exercise testing and recovery
- Absence of angina or other significant symptoms (*e.g.,* unusual shortness of breath, light-headedness, or dizziness, during exercise testing and recovery)
- Presence of normal hemodynamics during exercise testing and recovery (*i.e.,* appropriate increases and decreases in heart rate and systolic blood pressure with increasing workloads and recovery)
- Functional capacity ≥7 METs

Nonexercise Testing Findings

- Resting ejection fraction ≥50%
- Uncomplicated myocardial infarction or revascularization procedure
- Absence of complicated ventricular dysrhythmias at rest
- Absence of congestive heart failure
- Absence of signs or symptoms of postevent/postprocedure ischemia
- Absence of clinical depression

MODERATE RISK

Characteristics of patients at moderate risk for exercise participation (any one or combination of these findings places a patient at moderate risk)

- Presence of angina or other significant symptoms (*e.g.,* unusual shortness of breath, light-headedness, or dizziness occurring only at high levels of exertion [≥7 METs])
- Mild to moderate level of silent ischemia during exercise testing or recovery (ST-segment depression <2 mm from baseline)
- Functional capacity <5 METs

Nonexercise Testing Findings

- Rest ejection fraction = 40%–49%

HIGH RISK

Characteristics of patients at high risk for exercise participation (any one or combination of these findings places a patient at high risk)

- Presence of complex ventricular dysrhythmias during exercise testing or recovery
- Presence of angina or other significant symptoms (*e.g.,* unusual shortness of breath, light-headedness, or dizziness at low levels of exertion [<5 METs] or during recovery)
- High level of silent ischemia (ST-segment depression ≥2 mm from baseline) during exercise testing or recovery (*continued*)

TABLE 13.6 *(Continued)*

- Presence of abnormal hemodynamics with exercise testing (i.e., chronotropic incompetence or flat or decreasing systolic BP with increasing workloads) or recovery (i.e., severe postexercise hypotension)

Nonexercise Testing Findings

- Rest ejection fraction <40%
- History of cardiac arrest or sudden death
- Complex dysrhythmias at rest
- Complicated myocardial infarction or revascularization procedure
- Presence of congestive heart failure
- Presence of signs or symptoms of postevent/postprocedure ischemia
- Presence of clinical depression

Reprinted from Williams MA. Exercise testing in cardiac rehabilitation: exercise prescription and beyond. Cardiol Clin. 2001;19:415–431

rotic coronary artery disease is the overwhelming cause of exercise-related deaths in adults, accounting for one exertion-related death per year for every 15,000–18,000 seemingly healthy men (38). The relative risk of both exercise-related myocardial infarction and sudden death is most likely in individuals who are the least physically active and who engage in unaccustomed vigorous physical activity (38). Therefore, sedentary adults should avoid unaccustomed vigorous activity (should begin with low- or moderate-intensity exercise), and gradually increase their activity levels over time (37). Selected exercise testing should be performed at the discretion of the physician before vigorous exercise is recommended for patients with known cardiovascular problems, or for healthy men and women over the age of 45 and 55, respectively (38).

Treatment

The AHA Statement on Exercise and CVD (38) provides strong evidence supporting the use of exercise training in virtually all patients with cardiovascular disease. As stated in Chapter 3, such patients should undergo exercise testing prior to beginning an exercise program and should not engage in vigorous activity unless they have been cleared to do so by a cardiologist or other medical specialist.

The exercise component is a critical aspect of the rehabilitation process, reducing the likelihood of death, but not decreasing the incidence of nonfatal reinfarction (38). The reason for this is not yet known; however, there is some evidence to suggest that exercise training enhances electrical stability and reduces ventricular fibrillation or myocardial damage directly or via factors such as ischemic preconditioning (38). Table 13.7 highlights some of the addi-

---

TABLE 13.7 Benefits of Exercise Training in the Treatment of Specific CVD Conditions

---

1. *Heart failure:* exercise training can greatly improve effort tolerance and quality of life in these patients; although, there is no evidence of decreased morbidity and mortality.
2. *Myocardial infarction:* comprehensive, exercise-based cardiac rehabilitation reduces mortality rates, but does not reduce the risk of recurrent MI.
3. *Claudication and peripheral artery disease:* Exercise has been shown to improve walking distance. The greatest improvement with exercise training occurred when patients trained to maximal tolerated pain, when training lasted at least 6 months, and when walking was the primary mode of exercise.
4. *Angina pectoris:* Exercise training enhances quality of life and reduces the severity of symptoms by improving endothelial function and decreasing the heart rate response to exertion. Furthermore, exercise may serve as a primary therapy, particularly in patients who are not candidates for revascularization.

Source: Thompson et al, 2003

tional cardiovascular conditions in which exercise is an important component of treatment.

As we have just illustrated, exercise is an important part of the treatment of both acute and chronic cardiovascular conditions. For patients who have had an acute cardiovascular event (particularly coronary artery disease, cardiac valve replacement, or a myocardial infarction), exercise training should be initiated while the patient is still in the hospital, and should continue long after the patient is discharged—hopefully for life (2). There are, however, situations where exercise is contraindicated in patients with cardiovascular disease. Table 13.8 outlines both the indications and contraindications for exercise in cardiac patients.

Inpatient treatment should include early assessment and mobilization, identification of and education regarding CVD risk factors, assessment of the patient's level of readiness for physical activity, and comprehensive discharge planning. Exercise should be supervised with physiological monitoring, and progress should be slow, beginning with basic mobilization such as bed exercises, sitting at the bedside, and progressing to supervised walking on the ward.

Outpatient exercise training should begin soon after hospital discharge and should be clinically supervised. In addition, patients should be taught to identify abnormal signs and symptoms. Progression of exercise follows on from inpatient training, with continued gradual increases in exercise as tolerated. Table 13.9 outlines the recommended progression of exercise for cardiac patients.

TABLE 13.8 Clinical Indications and Contraindications for Cardiac Rehabilitation

Indications

- Medically stable post MI
- Stable angina
- Coronary artery bypass graft surgery (CABG)
- Percutaneous transluminal coronary angioplasty (PTCA) or other trans-catheter procedure
- Compensated congestive heart failure (CHF)
- Cardiomyopathy
- Heart or other organ transplantation
- Other cardiac surgery such as valvular and pacemaker insertion including implantable cardioverter defibrillator (ICD)
- Peripheral arterial disease (PAD)
- High-risk CVD ineligible for surgical intervention
- Sudden cardiac death syndrome
- End stage renal disease
- At risk for coronary artery disease with a diagnoses of diabetes mellitus, dyslipidemia, hypertension, obesity, or other diseases and conditions
- Other patients who may benefit from structured exercise and/or patient education based on physician referral and consensus of the rehabilitation team

Contraindications

- Unstable angina
- Resting systolic BP (SBP) >200 mm Hg or resting diastolic BP (DBP) >110 mm Hg that should be evaluated on a case by case basis
- Orthostatic BP drop of >20 mm Hg with symptoms
- Critical aortic stenosis (i.e., peak SBP gradient of >50 mm Hg with an aortic valve orifice area of <0.75 cm^2 in an average size adult)
- Acute systemic illness or fever
- Uncontrolled atrial or ventricular dysrhythmias
- Uncontrolled sinus tachycardia (>120 beats/min)
- Uncompensated CHF
- Third degree atrioventricular (AV) block without pacemaker
- Active pericarditis or myocarditis
- Recent embolism
- Thrombophlebitis
- Resting ST segment depression or elevation (>2 mm)
- Uncontrolled diabetes mellitus (DM) (see Chapter 13 for more on exercise and DM)
- Severe orthopedic conditions that would prohibit exercise
- Other metabolic conditions such as acute thyroiditis, hypokalemia, hyperkalemia, or hypovolemia.

(from: ACSM's Exercise prescription for patients with cardiac disease. In: American College of Sports Medicine. 8th ed. Philadelphia: Lippincott Williams & Wilkins. 2009. pp. 202–224.)

TABLE 13.9 Exercise Recommendations for Cardiac Patients

	No exercise or pharmacologic test available	Pharmacologic test available (negative for ischemia)	Pharmacologic test available (positive for ischemia)
Training HR	Upper limit of HR_{rest} + 20 beats/min. Gradually titrate to higher levels according RPE, signs and symptoms, normal physiologic responses.	If good HR increase: 70–85% HR_{max}. If HR does not increase: HR_{rest} + 20 beats/min with progression as described for no exercise or pharmacologic test available.	10 beats/min below ischemic threshold (if determined). If ischemic threshold not determined, use procedure for no exercise or pharmacologic test available.
Initial MET Level	2–4	2–4	2–4
Monitoring	ECG, BP, RPE, and signs or symptoms of ischemia	ECG, BP, RPE, and signs or symptoms of ischemia	ECG, BP, RPE, and signs or symptoms of ischemia
RPE (10pt scale)	3–5	3–5	3–5
MET Progression Increments	1–2	1–2	1–2

Initial workload of 2–4 METs is equivalent to Treadmill: 1.7 mph/0–7.5% grade; 2.0 mph/0–5.0% grade; 2.5 mph/0–2.5% grade; Leg Cycle Ergometry: ≤0 W; Arm Ergometry: ≤25 W

Progression of 1–2 METs is equivalent to Treadmill: 1–1.5 mph or 1–2% grade; Leg Cycle Ergometry: 25–50 W; and Arm Ergometry: ≤25 W

HR = heart rate; ECG = electrocardiogram; BP = blood pressure; RPE = rating of perceived exertion

Adapted from: ACSM's Exercise prescription for patients with cardiac disease. In: American College of Sports Medicine. 8th ed. Philadelphia: Lippincott Williams & Wilkins. 2009. pp. 202–224.

OLDER ADULTS

Advancing age increases the risk of developing and ultimately dying from many of the other conditions discussed in this chapter, including cardiovascular disease, type 2 diabetes, hypertension, and certain cancers. Moreover, older populations have the highest prevalence of degenerative conditions such as osteoporosis and arthritis. Therefore, your patient's exercise prescription will likely need to address any chronic illness as well as advancing age.

Regular physical activity including cardiovascular and resistance exercise is essential to healthy aging. The benefits of exercise in older adults improve functional capacity, chronic disease risk reduction, and quality of life.

It is important to recognize that healthy, sedentary older men and women have qualitatively similar physiological adjustments to exercise as young adults have (40). Although the absolute improvements tend to be less in older adults, the relative increases in aerobic and resistance training are similar, though perhaps take longer to achieve in older adults. For example, even frail, institutionalized older adults can substantially increase muscle strength with resistance exercises (41).

Illness or Condition

- While aging is not necessarily a pathologic state, "advancing age is associated with physiological changes that result in reductions in functional capacity and altered body composition" (42).

Definition

- When viewed as a developmental process, aging is lifelong. For purposes of formal exercise recommendations, "older adults" refers to individuals ≥65 years old, or those aged 50–64 with clinically significant medical conditions and/or functional limitations.

Prevalence and Incidence

- By 2030 it is estimated that more than 20% of the US population will be ≥65 years old, with the most rapidly expanding group those ≥85 years old. Older adults are the least physically active group (43). Yet, regular physical activity in the form of aerobic activity and muscle strengthening exercises is essential for healthy aging (44).

Other Treatments (Medication, Surgery, Etc.)

- There is, of course, no treatment for aging; however, sedentary behavior closely mimics the aging process, with resultant declines in physiologic measures such as declines in maximal aerobic capacity ($\dot{V}O2max$) and skeletal muscle performance. Exercise can slow these normal declines due to physiological aging and, therefore, preserve physical independence in older adults.

Further, regular exercise increases active life expectancy by limiting the development and progression of chronic disease and disabling conditions (42).

Testing and Screening

- As with younger adults, screening should not present a barrier to initiating physical activity due to the marked benefits of physical activity versus the small risks of injury. "For sedentary older people who are asymptomatic, low-intensity physical activity can be safely initiated regardless of whether or not an older person has had a recent medical evaluation" (45).

Precautions

- Older adults are more susceptible to heat and cold stress.

Exercise Prescription: Modifications From General Recommendations

- The physical activity recommendations of the ACSM/AHA referred to throughout the book are addressed to adults aged 15–65 years old. However, ACSM/AHA released simultaneously with these recommendations a companion paper addressing older adults (≥65 years old) (44). The exercise prescription for older adults should include cardiovascular exercise, resistance training, flexibility exercises, and specific exercises to improve balance in those at risk for falling (46) or those who have impaired mobility.

The most significant differences in the recommendations for exercise prescription in older adults are:

- Lower intensity of exercise: Vigorous-intensity exercise is not necessary to reduce the risks of developing chronic cardiovascular and metabolic disease (42). Low-intensity exercise is a reasonable starting point, especially for previously sedentary older adults. Moreover, progression to higher-intensity or longer periods of exercise may take several months. Higher-intensity exercise is, however, more effective in some illnesses and conditions such as diabetes, clinical depression, osteopenia, and muscle weakness. Due to the potentially low fitness levels in some older adults, exercise intensity should be measured in perceived exertion (see Chapter 8 for discussion of exercise intensity). For some previously sedentary older adults, a slow walk may be perceived as a high-intensity exertion.
- Going beyond minimal recommendations: As with younger adults, older patients should be encouraged to progress beyond the minimal recommendations to accumulate 30 minutes of moderate-intensity physical activity at least five days per week. This is especially significant to address illnesses that will respond to higher levels of intensity or longer periods of exercise, *e.g.,* obesity.
- Resistance exercise: The patient should perform 10–15 repetitions (rather than 8–12 repetitions) of 8–10 different major muscle groups at a moderate

5–6 on a 10-point scale, to high perceived exertion 7–8 on a 10-point scale. One to three sets of resistance exercise should be performed two to three times per week. Individualized or group instruction is preferable to learn proper form and technique for resistance exercises; however, the National Institutes of Aging has specific instructions and pictures (47).

- Flexibility exercises are recommended to address the usual decline in range of motion of the joints associated with aging. "To maintain the flexibility necessary for regular physical activity and daily life, older adults should perform activities that maintain or increase flexibility at least two days per week for at least 10 minutes each day" (44).

- Balance exercises are indicated for individuals at risk for falling. "To reduce the risk of injuries from falls, community-dwelling older adults with substantial risk of falls (*e.g.,* with frequent falls or mobility problems) should perform exercises that maintain or improve balance" (44). This may include dancing, Tai-Chi, or specific balance exercises; however, any physical activity (such as walking) will tend to improve balance.

- A combination of cardiovascular and resistance exercise is most effective in addressing the deleterious effects of a sedentary lifestyle.

- Particularly for older adults, the exercise prescription will be more effective if the overall program integrates social support, self-efficacy, active choices, health contracts, assurances of safety, and positive reinforcement (45).

DEPRESSION

There is substantial evidence showing that regular physical activity protects against the onset of depression symptoms and major depressive disorder. Participation in physical activity programs reduces depression symptoms in people diagnosed as depressed, in healthy adults, and in medical patients without psychiatric disorders regardless of age, gender, race/ethnicity, or medical condition (48).

Greater initial physical fitness predicts rapid recovery from depression (49). Personal fitness is positively associated with mental health and well-being.

Higher rates of depression accompany many of the chronic conditions (*e.g.,* cardiovascular disease, cancer, arthritis) discussed elsewhere in this chapter. These chronic conditions can be further complicated by weight gain from many psychiatric medications and by higher rates of smoking among patients with depression. The impaired motivation and low energy that often accompany depression interfere with the patient's ability to adhere to an exercise prescription. Yet, exercise is an effective treatment and preventive agent for mild to moderate depression.

In addition to the general health benefits of exercise, patients with depression and anxiety will experience improved sleep and improved glucose tolerance, which will counter the side effects of certain psychiatric medications and will allow patients an enhanced sense of self-efficacy ("taking control" of their illness).

The frequent monitoring by clinicians prescribing psychotropic medications presents an opportunity to prescribe exercise and reinforce the message through repeated visits.

Illness or Condition

• Depression ranges from minor chronic form, dysthymia, to the more severe form, major depressive disorder (MDD)

Definition

• The American Psychiatric Association (APA DSM-IV) defines Major Depressive Disorder in patients when they have a depressed mood or lose interest or pleasure in normal activities most of the time for at least two weeks. Other symptoms include abnormalities in appetite, libido, sleep, energy levels, concentration, and, often, suicidal thoughts.

Prevalence and Incidence

• Depression has an annual prevalence of about 8% in women and 4% in men in the United States and worldwide. The lifetime prevalence is about 16% (48).

Other Treatments

• Medications
• Electroconvulsive therapy
• Individual psychotherapy
• Group psychotherapy

"There is now considerable evidence that regular exercise is a viable, cost-effective but underused treatment for mild to moderate depression that compares favorably to individual psychotherapy, group psychotherapy, and cognitive therapy." (50)

Established Guidelines

• The United States Department of Health and Human Services Physical Activity Guidelines Advisory Committee Report addresses mental health and physical activity (48).

Precautions

• Physically healthy people who require psychotropic medication may safely exercise when exercise and medication are titrated under close medical supervision.

Exercise Prescription: Modifications From General Recommendations

- Depressed patients will require the same exercise prescription. Closer follow-up to ensure adherence is advisable.
- **Intensity:** Moderate and high levels of physical activity similarly reduce the odds of developing depression symptoms, compared to low levels of physical activity (48). Even at low levels of activity, physically active individuals have lower levels of depression compared to sedentary individuals (49).

DIABETES

Definition

Diabetes mellitus is a group of metabolic diseases characterized by an elevated fasting blood glucose level (*i.e.,* hyperglycemia) as a result of either defects in insulin secretion or an inability to use insulin. Sustained elevated blood glucose levels place patients at risk for micro- and macrovascular diseases as well as neuropathies (peripheral and autonomic).

Four types of diabetes are recognized, based on etiologic origin: type 1, type 2, gestational (*i.e.,* diagnosed during pregnancy, see Pregnancy section above), and other specific origins (*i.e.,* genetic defects and drug-induced). However, most patients (90% of all cases) have type 2, followed by type 1 (5–10% of all cases) (51).

Diabetes Mellitus is diagnosed with fasting plasma glucose >126 mg per dL (7.0 mmol per L), while pre-diabetes is diagnosed with 100 mg per dL (5.6 mmol per L) to 125 mg per dL (6.9 mmol per L) (51). Pre-diabetes is a risk factor for future diabetes mellitus and atherosclerotic cardiovascular disease (CVD).

Hypoglycemia is defined as blood glucose level <70 mg per dL (3.9 mmol per L).

Incidence and Prevalence

Currently, 7% of the United States population has diabetes mellitus, with 1.5 million new cases diagnosed each year (52).

Benefits of Exercise

- Improved glucose tolerance
- Increased insulin sensitivity
- Decreased HbA_{1C}
- Decreased insulin requirements
- Improvement in CVD risk factors, *i.e.,* lipid profiles, BP, body weight, functional capacity, and well-being (51).
- Prevention of type 2 diabetes mellitus in those considered at high risk (*i.e.,* pre-diabetic) for developing the disease

- A primary purpose for a person with type 1 diabetes mellitus to undertake an exercise program is often cardiovascular health/fitness-related; whereas, for a person with type 2 diabetes mellitus, the primary purposes are often healthy weight loss maintenance and improved glucose disposal[2].

Other Treatments

- Diet
- Insulin
- Oral hypoglycemic agents

Screening

Prior to beginning an exercise program, patients with diabetes mellitus should undergo an extensive medical evaluation, particularly of the cardiovascular, nervous, renal, and visual systems to identify related diabetic complications. (See Precautions below.)

If patients are asymptomatic for cardiovascular disease (and at low risk for cardiac events) they may begin an exercise program of low to moderate intensity, without exercise testing. (See Table 3.2) (53).

However, diabetic patients with a higher risk of cardiac events who want to initiate vigorous-intensity exercises should undergo a medically supervised graded exercise test (GXT) with electrographic (ECG) monitoring (51). (See Table 3.4.) If patients have an abnormal exercise ECG or cannot perform a GXT due to deconditioning, peripheral artery disease (PAD), orthopedic disabilities, or neurologic diseases, they may require a radionuclide stress test or stress echocardiography (51).

Autonomic neuropathy increases the likelihood of cardiovascular disease. Therefore, patients with autonomic neuropathy who wish to initiate or increase a physical activity should undergo a thorough cardiac screening, including thallium scintigraphy (54).

Current guidelines to detect CVD in patients with diabetes mellitus often fail to detect silent ischemia (55).

Consequently, annual cardiovascular risk factor identification should be conducted by a clinician (51).

Exercise Prescription

The general recommendations for exercise prescription apply to people with diabetes mellitus. Because of the marked overlap between diabetes and other medical conditions, such as overweight/obesity, cardiovascular disease, and hypertension, please see earlier sections of this chapter for other guidelines.

The *aerobic exercise* training prescription for those with diabetes mellitus:

Frequency: At least five days per week. Avoidance of two consecutive days of inactivity helps sustain the glucose lowering effects and improved insulin sensitivity from exercise. However, even minimal amounts of activity (*e.g.,* a single bout of 10 minutes of low- to moderate-intensity physical activity) has beneficial effects compared to sedentary behavior.

Intensity: Low-intensity physical activity is an appropriate starting place for previously sedentary patients with the goal of advancing to moderate-intensity physical activity. Progressing to vigorous activity will confer greater cardiovascular benefits, but with an increased risk and without significant additional benefits toward preventing or treating diabetes.

Time: The goal is 20 to 60 minutes of daily moderate-intensity physical activity accumulated in bouts of at least 10 minutes of activity. Patients should strive to accumulate a minimum of 1000 kcal per week (56) either through 150 minutes per week of moderate-intensity, or 90 minutes per week of vigorous-intensity, or some combination of moderate and vigorous-intensity physical activity for health/fitness benefits (51). Greater amounts of moderate-intensity exercise that result in a caloric energy expenditure of ≥ 2000 kcal per week, including daily exercise, may be required if weight-loss maintenance is the goal, as is the case for most people with type 2 diabetes mellitus (57).

Type: Emphasize activities that use large muscle groups in a rhythmic and continuous fashion. Personal interest and desired goals of the exercise program should be considered.

Resistance training may serve as a treatment for diabetes (58, 59) and should be encouraged for people with diabetes mellitus in the absence of contraindications, such as retinopathy and recent laser treatments. The recommendations for healthy persons generally apply to patients with diabetes mellitus:

Frequency: At least twice per week on non-consecutive days

Intensity: Two to three sets of eight to 12 repetitions to the point of volitional fatigue on the last repetition

Time: Eight to 10 multi-joint exercises of all major muscle groups in the same session (whole body) or sessions may be split into selected muscle groups

Type: Due to the likelihood of comorbidities such as hypertension, emphasize proper technique, including minimizing sustained gripping, static work, and the Valsalva maneuver to prevent an exacerbated blood pressure response.

Precautions

Hypoglycemia is a common problem in diabetic patients on insulin or oral hypoglycemic agents and who are exercising. Rapid drops in blood glucose may occur and produce symptoms even in elevated glycemic states. Hypoglycemia may be mitigated through blood glucose monitoring before and after exercise, especially on beginning or increasing an exercise program. Also, timing of exercise to avoid peak insulin action should be considered. Exercise with a partner or under supervision is recommended to reduce the risk of problems associated with hypoglycemic events.

Hyperglycemia, with or without ketosis, is a concern for people with type 1 diabetes mellitus who are not in glycemic control.

Polyuria, a common occurrence of hyperglycemia, may cause dehydration and contribute to a compromised thermoregulatory response (60). Thus, a patient with hyperglycemia should be treated as having an elevated risk for heat illness requiring more frequent monitoring of signs and symptoms.

Retinopathy increases the risk for retinal detachment and vitreous hemorrhage associated with vigorous-intensity exercise. Therefore, patients should avoid activities that dramatically elevate blood pressures. Patients with severe nonproliferative and proliferative diabetic retinopathy should avoid vigorous-intensity aerobic and resistance exercise (51, 54).

Autonomic neuropathy may affect heart rate response to exercise. Therefore, ratings of perceived exertion may be a more appropriate means of moderating the intensity of physical activity. Autonomic neuropathy may also blunt the systolic blood pressure response, attenuate $\dot{V}O2$ kinetics and anhydrosis (51, 60). Therefore, monitor the signs and symptoms of hypoglycemia and silent ischemia, because of the inability of the patient to recognize them. Also monitor blood pressure following exercise to manage hypotension and hypertension associated with vigorous-intensity exercise (60). Autonomic neuropathy may also impair thermoregulation in hot and cold environments (51); therefore, additional precautions for heat and cold illness are warranted.

Peripheral neuropathy and/or diabetic foot problems may limit walking and require nonweight-bearing exercises. Careful foot care to avoid blisters and ulcers is important.

Nephropathy does not preclude vigorous exercise, although protein excretion acutely increases postexercise. There is no evidence that vigorous-intensity exercise accelerates the rate of progression of kidney disease (51).

References

1. Durstine JL, Moore GE, editors. ACSM's exercise management for persons with chronic disease and disability book. 2nd ed. Champaign (IL): Human Kinetics; 2003. 374 p.

Arthritis

2. Multiple Authors. Exercise prescription for other clinical populations. In: Thompson WR, senior editor, Gordon NF, Pescatello LS, associate editors. ACSM's guidelines for exercise testing and prescription. 8th ed. Philadelphia (PA): Lippincott Williams & Wilkins; 2009. p. 225–272.

3. Centers for Disease Control and Prevention (US). Prevalence of disabilities and associated health conditions among adults: United States, 1999. Morb Mortal Wkly Rep. 2001 Feb 23;50(7):120–5.

4. Centers for Disease Control and Prevention (US). Prevalence of doctor-diagnosed arthritis and arthritis related activity limitation: United States, 2003–2005. Morb Mortal Wkly Rep. 2006 Oct 12;55(40):1089–92.

5. Wilkins A, Phillips E. Osteoarthritis. In: Frontera WF, Silver J, Rizzo TD Jr, editors. Essentials of physical medicine and rehabilitation: musculoskeletal disorders, pain, and rehabilitation. 2nd ed. Philadelphia (PA): Saunders; 2008. p. 745–751.

Hypertension

6. Chobanian AV, Bakris GL, Black HR, Cushman WC, Green LA, Izzo JL Jr, Jones DW, Materson BJ, Oparil S, Wright JT Jr, Roccella EJ; Joint National Committee on Prevention, Detection, Evaluation, and Treatment of High Blood Pressure (US); National Heart, Lung, and Blood Institute (US); National High Blood Pressure Education Program Coordinating Committee (US). The seventh report of the Joint National Committee on Prevention, Detection, Evaluation, and Treatment of High Blood Pressure. Hypertension. 2003 Dec;42(6):1206–52.
7. Pescatello LS, Franklin BA, Fagard R, Farquhar WB, Kelley GA, Ray CA; American College of Sports Medicine (US). American College of Sports Medicine position stand. Exercise and hypertension. Med Sci Sports Exerc. 2004 Mar;36(3):533–53.

Overweight and Obesity

8. Ogden CL, Carroll MD, Curtin LR, McDowell MA, Tabak CJ, Flegal KM. Prevalence of overweight and obesity in the United States, 1999–2004. JAMA. 2006 Apr; 295(13):1549–55.
9. National Institute of Health (US); National Heart, Lung, and Blood Institute (US). Clinical guidelines on the identification, evaluation, and treatment of overweight and obesity in adults: the evidence report. Obes Res. 1998 Sep;6(suppl. 2):S51–209.
10. Wing RR. Behavioral weight control. In: Wadden TA, Stunkard AJ, editors. Handbook of obesity treatment. New York: The Guilford Press; 2002. p. 301–16.
11. U.S. Department of Health and Human Services; US Department of Agriculture. Dietary guidelines for Americans, 2005 [Internet]. 6th ed. Washington (DC): US Government Printing Office; 2005 Jan [cited 2008 Oct 4]. Available from: http://www.health.gov/dietaryguidelines/dga2005/document/default.htm
12. Bren L. Losing weight: start by counting calories. FDA Consumer Mag [Internet]. 2002 Jan-Feb [revised 2002 Apr, 2003 Mar, 2004 Apr; cited 2008 Jul 17];36(1):[8 p.]. Available from: http://www.fda.gov/FDAC/features/2002/102_fat.html

Osteoporosis

13. Kohrt WM, Bloomfield SA, Little KD, Nelson ME, Yingling VR. American College of Sports Medicine position stand: physical activity and bone health. Med Sci Sport Exerc. 2004 Mon;36(11):1985–96.
14. Kanis JA, Melton LJ, Christiansen C, Johnston CC, Khaltaev N. The diagnosis of osteoporosis. J Bone Miner Res. 1994 Aug;9(8):1137–41.
15. Binkley N, Bilezikian JP, Kendler DL, Leib ES, Lewiecki EM, Petak SM. Official positions of the International Society for Clinical Densitometry and executive summary of the 2005 Position Development Conference. J Clin Densitom. 2006 Jan-Mar;9(1):4–14.
16. Hans D, Downs RW, Duboeuf F, Greenspan S, Jankowski LG, Kiebzak GM, Petak SM. Skeletal sites for osteoporosis diagnosis: the 2005 ISCD Official Positions. J Clin Densitom. 2006 Jan-Mar;9(1):15–21.
17. US Department of Health and Human Services. Bone health and osteoporosis: a report of the Surgeon General. Rockville (MD): U.S. Department of Health and Human Services, Office of the Surgeon General; 2004. 436 p.
18. Beck BR, Snow CM. Bone health across the lifespan: exercising our options. Exerc Sport Sci Rev. 2003 Jul;31(3):117–22.

19. Robertson MC, Campbell AJ, Gardner MM, Devlin N. Preventing injuries in older people by preventing falls: a meta-analysis of individual-level data. J Am Geriatr Soc. 2002 May;50(5):905–11.
20. Sinaki M. The role of physical activity in bone health: a new hypothesis to reduce risk of vertebral fracture. Phys Med Rehabil Clin N Am. 2007 Aug;18(3):593–608.

Pregnancy
21. Petersen AM, Leet TL, Brownson RC. Correlates of physical activity among pregnant women in the United States. Med Sci Sport Exerc. 2005;37:1748–53.
22. Thompson D. Fitness Focus copy-and-share: exercise during pregnancy. ACSM'S Health & Fitness J. 2007 Mar/Apr;11(2):4.
23. O'Toole ML. Physiological aspects of exercise in pregnancy. Clin Obstet Gynecol. 2003;46:79–389.
24. Wolfe LA, Davies GAL. Canadian guidelines for exercise in pregnancy. Clin Obstet Gynecol. 2003;46:488–95.
25. Wolfe LA, Hall P, Webb KA et al. Prescription of aerobic exercise during pregnancy. Sports Med. 1989 Nov;8(5):273–301.
26. American Diabetes Association (US). Nutrition recommendations and interventions for diabetes: a position statement of the American Diabetes Association. Diabetes Care. 2007 Jan;30(Suppl 1):S48–S65.
27. Downs DS, Ulbrecht JS. Understanding exercise beliefs and behaviors in women with gestational diabetes mellitus. Diabetes Care. 2006 Feb;29(2):236–40.
28. Committee on Obstetric Practice, American College of Obstetricians and Gynecologists (US). ACOG committee opinion: exercise during pregnancy and the postpartum period. Obstet Gynecol. 2002 Jan;77(267):79–81.
29. Artal R, O'Toole M. Guidelines of the American College of Obstetricians and Gynecologists for exercise during pregnancy and the postpartum period. Br J Sports Med. 2003 Feb;37(1):6–12.
30. Artal R, Sherman C. Exercise during pregnancy. Phys Sports Med. 1999 Mon;27(#):51.
31. Soultanakis-aligianni HN. Thermoregulation during exercise in pregnancy. Clin Obstet Gynecol. 2003 Jun;46(2):442–55.
32. Katz VL. Exercise in water during pregnancy. Clin Obstet Gynecol. 2003;46:432–41.
33. Dumoulin C. Postnatal pelvic floor muscle training for preventing and treating urinary incontinence: where do we stand? Clin Obstet Gynecol. 2006 Oct;18(5):538–43.
34. American Diabetes Association. Position statement: gestational diabetes mellitus. Diabetes Care. 2004 Jan;27(Suppl 1): S88–S90.

Cancer
35. American Cancer Society (US). Cancer facts and figures 2006. Atlanta (GA): American Cancer Society (US); 2006. Available from: http://www.cancer.org/downloads/STT/CAFF_2006_PW_secured.pdf
36. Ness KK, Wall MM, Oakes JM, Robison LL, Gurney JG. Physical performance limitations and participation restrictions among cancer survivors: a population-based study. Ann Epidemiol. 2006 Mar;16(5):197–205.

Cardiovascular Disease
37. Thompson PD. Exercise and physical activity in the prevention and treatment of atherosclerotic cardiovascular disease. Arterioscler Thromb Vasc Biol. 2003 Aug;23(5):1319–21.

38. Thompson PD, Buchner D, Pina IL, Balady GJ, Williams MA, Marcus BH, Berra K, Blair SN, Costa F, Franklin B, Fletcher GF, Gordon NF, Pate RR, Rodriguez BL, Yancey AK, Wenger NK. Exercise and physical activity in the prevention and treatment of atherosclerotic cardiovascular disease: a statement from the Council on Clinical Cardiology (Subcommittee on Exercise, Rehabilitation, and Prevention) and the Council on Nutrition, Physical Activity, and Metabolism (Subcommittee on Physical Activity). Circulation. 2003 Jun;107(24):3109–16.

39. Fletcher GF, Balady GJ, Amsterdam EA, Chaitman B, Eckel R, Fieg J, Froelicher VF. Exercise standards for testing and training: a statement for healthcare professionals from the American Heart Association. Circulation. 2001 Oct;104(14):1694–740.

Older Adults

40. Seals DR, Taylor JA, Ng AV, Esler MD. Exercise and aging: autonomic control of the circulation. Med Sci Sports Exerc. 1994 May;26(5):568–76.

41. Fiatarone MA, Marks EC, Ryan ND, Meredith CN, Lipsitz LA, Evan WJ. High intensity strength training in nonagenarians: effects on skeletal muscle. JAMA. 1990 Jun;263(22):3029–34.

42. Chodzko-Zajko W, Minson CT, Nigg CR, Fiatarone Singh MA, Proctor D, Salem GJ, Skinner JS. ACSM position stand on exercise and physical activity for older adults. 2009.

43. Centers for Disease Control and Prevention (US). Prevalence of physical activity, including lifestyle activities among adults: United States, 2000–2001. MMWR Morb Mortal Wkly Rep. 2003 Aug 15;52(32):764–9.

44. Nelson ME, Rejeski WJ, Blair SN, Duncan PW, Judge JO, King AC, Macera CA, Castaneda-Sceppa C. Physical activity and public health in older adults: recommendation from the American College of Sports Medicine and the American Heart Association. Med Sci Sports Exerc. 2007 Aug;39(8):1435–45.

45. Cress ME, Buchner DM, Prohaska T, Rimmer J, Brown M, Macera C, DePietro L, Chodzko-Zajko W. Best practices for physical activity programs and behavioral counseling in older adults populations. J Aging Phys Act. 2005 Jan;13(1):61–74.

46. American Geriatrics Society (US); British Geriatrics Society (UK); and American Academy of Orthopaedic Surgeons Panel on Falls Prevention (US). Guideline for the prevention of falls in older persons. J Am Geriatr Soc. 2001 May;49(5):664–72.

47. National Institute on Aging (US). Exercise: a guideline from the National Institute on Aging. Bethesda (MD): National Institute on Aging (US); 1998. 88 p. Report No. NIH 98-4258. Available without charge through NIA Public Information Office (US) at 1-800-222-2225. [See resource list.]

Depression

48. Office of Disease Prevention and Health Promotion (US). Physical Activity Guidelines Advisory Committee Report [Internet]. Rockville (MD): U.S. Department of Health and Human Services; c2008 [revised 2008 Jun 11]. Part G, Section 8, Mental health; [cited 2008 Jul 18]; 32 p. Available from: http://www.health.gov/PAguidelines/Report/G8_mentalhealth.aspx

49. Morgan WP. Physical activity, fitness and depression. In: Bouchard C, Shephard RJ, Stevens T, editors. Physical activity, fitness, and health. Champaign (IL): Human Kinetics; 1994. p. 851–67.

50. Tkachuck GA, Martin GL. Exercise therapy for patients with psychiatric disorders: research and clinical implications. Prof Psychol Res and Pract. 1999 Jun;30(3): 275–82.

Diabetes

51. American Diabetes Association (US). Standards of medical care in diabetes 2007. Diabetes Care. 2007 Jan;30(Suppl 1):S4-S41.

52. Centers for Disease Control and Prevention (US). National diabetes fact sheet: general information and national estimates on diabetes in the United States, 2005 [Internet]. Atlanta (GA): U.S. Department of Health and Human Services, Centers for Disease Control and Prevention; c2006 [cited 2008 Oct 3]. 10 p. Available from: http://www.cdc.gov/diabetes/pubs/pdf/ndfs_2005.pdf

53. U.S. Preventive Task Force (US). Screening for coronary artery disease: recommendations statement. Ann Intern Med. 2004 Apr;140(7):569–72.

54. Sigal RJ, Kenny GP, Wasserman DH, Castaneda-Sceppa C, White RD. Physical activity/exercise and type 2 diabetes: A consensus statement from the American Diabetes Association. Diabetes Care. 2006 Jun;29(6):1433–8.

55. Wackers FJ, Young LH, Inzucchi SE, Chyun DA, Davey JA, Barrett EJ, Taillefer R, Wittlin SD, Heller GV, Filipchuk N, Engel S, Ratner RE, Iskandrian AE. Detection of ischemia in asymptomatic diabetics investigators: detection of silent myocardial ischemia in asymptomatic diabetic subjects: the DIAD study. Diabetes Care. 2004 Aug;27(8):1954–61.

56. Albright A, Franz M, Hornsby G, Kriska A, Marrero D, Ullrich I, Verity LS. American College of Sports Medicine position stand: exercise and type 2 diabetes. Med Sci Sports Exerc. 2000 Jul;32(7):1345–60.

57. American College of Sports Medicine (US). Position stand: appropriate intervention strategies for weight loss and prevention of weight regain for adults. Med Sci Sports Exerc. 2001 Dec;33(12):2145–56.

58. Dunstan DW, Daly RM, Owen N, Jolley D, De Court, Shaw J, Zimmet P. High-intensity resistance training improves glycemic control in older patients with type 2 diabetes. Diabetes Care. 2002 Oct;25(10):1729–36.

59. Sigal RJ, Kenny GP, Boule NG, Wells GA, Prud'homme D, Fortier M, Reid RD, Tulloch H, Coyle D, Phillips P, et al. Effects of aerobic training, resistance training, or both on glycemic control in type 2 diabetes: a randomized trial. Ann Intern Med. 2007 Sep;147(6):357–69.

60. Vinik A, Erbas T. Neuropathy. In: Ruderman N, Devlin JT, Schneider SH, Kriska A, editors. Handbook of exercise in diabetes. 2nd ed. Alexandria (VA): American Diabetes Association (US); 2002. p. 463–496.

CHAPTER 14

Exercise in Children: "Exercise is a Family Affair"

Evonne Kaplan-Liss and Mary Ellen Renna

INTRODUCTION

As noted throughout this book, the hard part of regular exercise is the "regular" and not the exercise. This is even truer for the pediatric population than it is for the adult population. Children are dependent on the family unit; therefore, the best chance of incorporating regular exercise into their daily lives is by making exercise a family affair. The goal of this chapter is to provide guidance to clinicians on how to counsel their pediatric patients and their families on making *exercise a family affair*.

This chapter discusses the importance of exercise in the pediatric population and the benefits of exercise to the entire family. The 5 As, as discussed in Chapter 2 (pp. 20–21; see also below), can be very helpful in organizing your intervention for this population. Let us recall them here: The "Five A's Framework:" **A**ssess, **A**dvise, **A**gree, **A**ssist, **A**rrange follow-up. They provide guidance on how you can effectively communicate the content of the American College of Sports Medicine's (ACSM) children and adolescent guidelines for physical activity at various stages of a child's development. The importance of the "new vital signs" (BMI measurements and exercise history) is stressed in this chapter and the barriers to regular family exercise are addressed. The ACSM Guidelines for the Exercise Prescription for Children and Adolescents are presented below (see pp. 232–233). They are designed to aid you in offering an exercise program that families can easily incorporate into their daily lives without the need for purchasing expensive equipment and freeing up a large amount of time. In order to ensure that regular exercise becomes a part of every family's daily routine, as we have said throughout this book, it will be very helpful for you to use each patient encounter to reinforce the message that "Exercise **IS** Medicine."

THE BENEFITS OF PHYSICAL ACTIVITY IN CHILDREN

The first step in counseling families to incorporate regular exercise into their daily routine is to inform each family about the health benefits of regular exercise, as well as about the risks associated with lack of exercise. As stated in the

ACSM's Guidelines for Exercise Testing and Prescription (1), most *children* (defined as <13 yr) participate in adequate amounts of physical activity. Recent trends, however, show physical activity levels decreasing through adolescence (defined as 13–18 yr or Tanner Stage 5), such that the majority of adolescents are not participating in sufficient amounts of physical activity to meet recommended guidelines (2, 3). Physical activity, however, has been shown to reduce death rates from heart disease, colon cancer, hypertension and diabetes (4).

As noted for children as well as for adults, the prevalence of physical activity has declined, while the prevalence of obesity has increased. Data from two NHANES surveys (1976–1980 and 2003–2004) show that the prevalence of obesity has almost tripled in all age groups: for children aged 2–5 years, prevalence increased from 5.0% to 13.9%; for those aged 6–11 years, prevalence increased from 6.5% to 18.8%; and for those aged 12–19 years, prevalence increased from 5.0% to 17.4% (5). Risk factors for cardiovascular disease (*i.e.,* elevated total cholesterol, triglycerides, insulin level, and blood pressure) and Type 2 Diabetes are more common in obese children than in those of normal weight. The obesity epidemic may potentially reverse the improved life expectancy trend that has resulted from the decrease in infectious diseases during the twentieth century; today's children may in fact have a shorter life expectancy than their parents (4). As is well-known, overweight children and adolescents are more likely to become obese adults, underscoring the magnitude of this public health problem. According to the Centers for Disease Control and Prevention (CDC), 80% of children who are overweight at 10–15 years of age are obese at age 25 (5).

It is clear that obesity has both genetic and environmental components. The environmental component is the well-known "more energy going in than being expended" factor. Clinicians may not be able to alter the genetic contribution to obesity, but they can influence the environmental contribution through nutritional and exercise counseling. (Nutrition counseling is beyond the scope of this chapter, but refer to *Growing Up Healthy* [7] for advice on nutrition counseling.)

Just as for adults, in addition to decreasing the risk for developing obesity and the co-morbidities associated with obesity (hypertension, heart disease, type II diabetes, arthritis, cardiomyopathy, fatty liver, and elevated triglycerides,) regular exercise in children has many other health benefits: improves bone density, especially in pre-pubertal children, helps to reduce future risk of osteoporosis, improves premenstrual syndrome, helps to reduce LDL cholesterol, and increases the heart-beneficial HDL cholesterol. Regular exercise also helps to improve muscle tone, strength, balance, and coordination.

Regular exercise has psychosocial benefits for children as well. Self-esteem improves in children who are physically active; school performance is enhanced; energy level is increased; and the risk of depression decreases through exercise's affects on hormonal levels (8, 9). In fact, because of the amelioration of some mood disorders with regular exercise, the exercise prescription is used by many pediatric psychiatrists to help alleviate symptoms in their patients (10). Children who are not physically active have a greater tendency to have depression and spend more time on computers, watching television, or playing video games than those who are physically active. These solitary and sedentary activities are obviously not conducive to developing a positive family environment (10). If children are engaging in regular exercise, overall harmony of the family can and will improve.

ACSM GUIDELINES FOR EXERCISE PRESCRIPTION FOR CHILDREN AND ADOLESCENTS (1)

Guidelines

ACSM's exercise prescription guidelines outlined below for children and adolescents establish the minimal amount of physical activity needed to achieve the various components of health-related fitness (11).

Frequency: most days of the week, and preferably daily.

Intensity: moderate (physical activity that *noticeably* increases breathing, sweating, and HR) to vigorous (physical activity that *substantially* increases breathing, sweating, and HR) intensity.

Time: 30 minutes of moderate and 30 minutes of vigorous intensity to total 60 minutes of accumulated physical activity.

Type: a variety of activities that are enjoyable and developmentally appropriate for the child or adolescent: Activities may include walking, active play/games, dance, and sports.

As for adults, children can be encouraged to engage in either lifestyle/activities of daily living or scheduled leisure-time regular exercise or both in some combination.

Special Considerations

- Children and adolescents may safely participate in strength-training activities, provided that they receive proper instruction and supervision. Generally, adult guidelines for resistance training may be applied. Eight to 15 repetitions of an exercise should be performed to the point of moderate fatigue with good mechanical form before the resistance is increased.
- Because of immature thermoregulatory systems, children and adolescents should exercise in thermoneutral environments and be properly hydrated. Refer to ACSM position stands on exercising in the heat (12) and fluid replacement (13) for additional information.

- Children and adolescents who are overweight or physically inactive may not be able to achieve 60 consecutive minutes of physical activity. Therefore, gradually increase the frequency and time of physical activity to achieve this goal.
- Children and adolescents with diseases or disabilities such as asthma, diabetes mellitus, obesity, cystic fibrosis, and cerebral palsy should have their exercise prescriptions tailored to their condition, symptoms, and functional capacity. Refer to Chapter 10 of *ACSM's Guidelines for Exercise Testing and Prescription* (1) for additional information on exercise recommendations for these diseases and conditions.
- Efforts should be made to decrease sedentary activities (*i.e.,* television watching, surfing the Internet, and playing video games) and increase activities that promote lifelong activity and fitness (*i.e.,* walking and cycling).

EXERCISE COUNSELING AND PRESCRIPTION

Each pediatric patient encounter provides an opportunity for you to recommend regular exercise for both your patient(s) and the whole family unit. Whether the office visit is a sick or well visit, it presents an opportunity for you to ask about exercise and nutrition habits. The well visit will beneficially incorporate the measurement of "the new vital signs," calculation of BMI and plotting of BMI percentile, as well as asking about the family's level of physical activity. Using the "5 As" (Assess, Advise, Agree, Assist, Arrange [see Chap. 2, pp. 20–21]) can help in organizing your counseling of the family on regular exercise. Since children are "not just small adults," it is important for you to take into consideration the developmental stage of the child or adolescent and alter the exercise prescription accordingly. Children and adolescents require special consideration when exercising as a result of growth and the immaturity of their physiologic regulatory systems at rest and during exercise. Physiologic responses to acute exercise are also different in children as compared to adults (see Table 14.1).

THE NEW VITAL SIGNS: BMI AND LEVEL OF PHYSICAL ACTIVITY

In order for you to begin incorporating regular exercise counseling into your practice, it is important to start by including "the new vital signs" in their routine vital sign screening and to learn how to interpret them. The "new vital signs" include measurement of body mass index (BMI) and level of physical activity. BMI is a measure of the weight in kilograms divided by the height in meters squared. A normal BMI based on age and sex falls between the fifth and 85th percentile when plotted on standardized BMI growth charts (14). BMI should be routinely measured and plotted at all yearly well visits. If the BMI plots above the 85th percentile, closer follow-up may be indicated.

TABLE 14.1 Physiologic Responses to Acute Exercise of Children Compared to Adults

Variable	
Absolute Oxygen Uptake ($\dot{V}O_2$ (L·min-1))	Lower
Relative Oxygen Uptake ($\dot{V}O_2$ (mL·kg·min-1))	Higher
Heart Rate	Higher
Cardiac Output	Lower
Stroke Volume	Lower
Systolic Blood Pressure	Lower
Diastolic Blood Pressure	Lower
Respiratory Rate	Higher
Tidal Volume	Lower
Minute Ventilation ($\dot{V}E$)	Lower
Respiratory Exchange Ratio	Lower

Adapted from Hebestreit HU, Bar-Or O. Differences between children and adults for exercise testing and prescription. In: Skinner JS, editor. Exercise testing and exercise prescription for special cases. Philadelphia (PA): Lippincott Williams & Wilkins; 2005. 68–84 p. and Strong WB, Malina RM, Blimke CJR, Daniels SR, Dishman RK, Gutin B, Hergenroeder AC, Must A, Nixon PA, Pivarnik JM, Rowland T, Trost S, Trudeau F. Evidence-based physical activity for school-age youth. J Pediatrics; 2005 Mon;146(__):732–7.

BMI ranges plotted on standardized curves:

	Healthy range	Overweight	Obese	Underweight
BMI kg/m²	5% to less than 85%	85% to less than 95%	>=95%	<5%

During every office visit, the clinician should take the opportunity to ask the patient and their present family member(s) about their exercise routine. This kind of inquiry reinforces the importance of exercise as a health promotive/disease preventive activity that both patient and family members can take.

THE 5 As

After measuring the "the new vital signs," the next step is to use the 5 As (Assess, Advise, Agree, Assist, Arrange) to prescribe regular exercise to each patient and her family, thereby ensuring that each family learns the key elements to making regular exercise a part of their daily lives. There are many issues you need to address during the well-child examination, with less and less time to go over all of them thoroughly. It is imperative that information about exercise and nutrition habits is obtained during this time. Asking key questions while performing the examination will save time and, if needed, a follow-up visit can be arranged for the families that need more guidance.

ASSESS

The assessment of each child's ability to participate in regular exercise starts with evaluating the child's overall health. Begin with a thorough family history and, as you do for diseases and negative health conditions, revisit the subject periodically thereafter for updates. A family history of sudden deaths with exercise, arrhythmias, renal diseases, or congenital abnormalities may lead to further evaluation. Beginning at age 3, well visits should include height, weight, BMI, BMI percentile, vision screen, and blood pressure. The physical exam should be a detailed well-child examination, including scoliosis screening. Laboratory work should include a hemoglobin and hematocrit in children with a history of anemia or risk for anemia. Lipid profiles should be done in children with family histories of hypercholesterolemia.

At the present time, the U.S. Preventive Services Task Force (USPSTF) recommends against routine screening with resting electrocardiography (ECG) for the prediction of coronary heart disease (CHD) events in adults at low risk for CHD events (15). Though no such recommendation has been issued for or against screening ECG in children, it is important to consider a full cardiac evaluation before recommending regular exercise for children with a history of fainting, irregular heart beat, or a family history of sudden death, cardiomyopathy, prolonged QT syndromes, or Marfan syndrome. The musculoskeletal exam assesses overall flexibility, tone, and joint inflammation. If inflammation is found on examination, it is important to postpone regular exercise until the inflammation resolves.

There are special circumstances to consider when dealing with chronically ill children as well as developmentally delayed children. The chronically ill child must have the disease under control before beginning regular exercise. For example, physical activity must be taken into account when determining insulin dose in children with diabetes. The asthmatic child must have pulmonary function levels in normal range before, during, and after exercise. The developmentally delayed child needs to have strict supervision with exercise. They also may also be more resistant to the exercise routine, so it is imperative that the activity is fun, stimulating, and rewarding for the child. This applies to all children, but carries more significance in developmentally delayed children.

The ability to understand that exercise contributes to health and well-being is more difficult for developmentally delayed children. Behavior problems may exist that may preclude the child's ability to engage in regular exercise. Despite the challenges in this pediatric population, it is even more worthwhile to remind the parents that exercise *IS* medicine, because regular exercise often improves the underlying medical condition as these children tend to be less physically fit because their medical conditions have prevented them from incorporating regular exercise into their daily routine. Many children want to please their doctor, and a constant reminder by the clinician to exercise may motivate the most stubborn child. (Refer to chapter 10 of *ACSM's Guidelines for Exercise Testing and Prescription* [1] for additional information on exercise recommendations for these diseases and conditions.)

ADVISE

The clinician is in the unique position to know a child and the family on all levels. They know the family history, medical history of the child, and the personality and development of the child, as well as the physical examination findings of the child. This information is useful when advising the family about regular exercise that is best suited for the child and the family.

The recommended exercise program is best developed with the level of muscle tone (low tone, normal tone, or high tone) in mind (16). Most children have normal tone; therefore, activity is unrestricted. In order to improve strength, balance, and coordination, the low-tone children benefit from single-activity resistance training like karate or Tae Kwon-Do. The high-tone children need to ease into a regular exercise program with careful maneuvers that will not cause physical damage. These children do better with swimming or calisthenics. Children with tight muscle tone (17) are more prone to injury, and therefore require careful attention to flexibility when exercising, emphasizing slow exercise and stretching; physical therapists or athletic trainers are often helpful when starting these children on their road to regular exercise.

The physical abilities and development of the child also needs to be taken into consideration when recommending an exercise regimen. The young child is obviously not able to engage in long-distance running; however, they may be able to ride a bike. The younger child exercises in the playground; whereas, the teenager will not engage in this activity for exercise and may require more structured regular exercise.

Anticipating that regular exercise will become a part of a child's daily routine is the key step to successful habit forming in this arena. It is important to teach parents at each visit, starting with the newborn visit, to incorporate regular exercise into their child's daily routine. Parents should be advised to start to exercise with their baby and gradually bring them into the routine as a family. Talk to parents about reducing television time, video game time, and computer time. Restricting these sedentary activities allows more time for the child to engage in physical activity and to socialize with the family. Each office visit is an opportunity to communicate to the parents that regular exercise for their children is best undertaken as a *family affair.*

If you are a regular exerciser yourself, it will help in convincing families about the importance of incorporating regular exercise into their daily routine. Children are very intuitive and will recognize if they are being told to do something by an adult who is not following their own advice. Talk to families about the activities that you like to do to keep fit. This helps put everyone on equal ground and will provide a role model for your patients and their families.

AGREE

Agree that it can be difficult to maintain a regular exercise program. Validating the feelings of the parents is a crucial step in helping them get into healthy habits. Recounting your own stories of the difficulties encountered with finding the will and time to exercise, but at the same time telling the parents and the child that it can be done, can be very helpful. Ask the child about the types of physical activities he likes to do. Validate and praise the child for participating in the activities and, if necessary, make some suggestions to improve on them.

ASSIST

Assist the parents and child in deciding what exercises, sports, or gym classes are best for the child. You might want to print out the exercise routine in this chapter (see, p. 243) and use it as a handout for your patients. This routine does not require any equipment and can be done anywhere. Make regular exercise as easy as possible for your patients. It is always easier for the parent if the exercise does not require special equipment or a car ride to a sports class. If the parent has the ability to pay for classes and the time to take their children to the class, this is a perfectly good adjunct to regular exercise; however, it is very important that children learn how to exercise *without* equipment, a sports team, or a class instructor. Making sure that a home exercise routine is always in place is a step to ensuring that regular exercise is a part of the child's life.

You can be very helpful in assisting your patients and their families in overcoming barriers to exercising regularly.

1. *Not enough time in the day to exercise.* Time for exercise can be more easily found if you recommend starting off with small bites of time. Recommend starting off with 10 minutes of short bursts of exercise three times a day to start.
2. *Too tired to exercise.* Help families to learn that exercise will only increase energy and lack of exercise contributes to feelings of fatigue.
3. *Don't know what types of exercise my child should be doing.* Any type of activity that gets a child running, jumping, or resistance training will work. Parents should know what is going on in their child's physical education

class and reinforce what they are learning in the home setting. Knowing what activities your child enjoys most during recess and playground time can also help you develop your child's exercise habits.

4. *Exercise is going to hurt my child.* There is a misconception that exercising is harmful to young children and should not be done. Children are never too young to exercise. A child who can run and jump is exercising. Young children will exercise within their developmental ability and will not hurt themselves, as long as there is proper supervision so that physical dangers are avoided.

5. *Exercising may affect growth negatively or cause bone damage.* It is a misconception that resistance training in children will cause permanent damage to growth (1). Resistance training can enhance all exercise routines and should be actively encouraged by the clinician. There is no danger to the growth plate when resistance training is done properly. This can include resistance training using the child's body weight (*e.g.*, push ups, pull ups, sit ups, etc.), or using weight training under the ACSM guidelines mentioned above (18). Many parents do not realize how beneficial resistance training is for children, and the clinician should educate the parents on the advantages to the growing skeleton, in particular the decreased risk for osteoporosis in the future (19, 20, 21).

ARRANGE

Arrange for follow-up. The best time for the clinician to present the exercise prescription for the first time is during a well visit, because there is more time to spend counseling patients then than at sick visits, but it is important to follow up at all visits, if at all possible. The family's reaction to the exercise prescription may be mixed, ranging from a good reception to the exercise recommendation to making excuses as to why they do not participate in regular exercise. The families that require closer follow-up are the families that verbalize the excuses to avoid following your recommendations. The more excuses, the more imperative becomes the follow-up visit. The families that are willing to listen and adhere to your recommendations need follow-up, but not necessarily a scheduled visit just for this purpose. All families can be followed up at any visit to the doctor's office. As stated above, you can ask the patient about how their exercise routine is going when they come in for a vaccine or if they come in for a fever.

EXERCISE PRESCRIPTION BY AGE

Obviously, clinicians deal with children at all stages of development. Therefore, you will want to approach the family and patient and adapt the exercise prescription according to these developmental stages.

Birth–Three Years

The first year of life offers many opportunities for you to stress the importance of preventive services like immunizations and regular exercise. Preventive services are always a tough sell, because they do not have apparent immediate health effects. Therefore, it is even more important to revisit these services at every opportunity. The prenatal and first postnatal office visits are the best times to start educating the parents on the importance of eating a healthy diet and how exercise can improve their life as well as their child's life. These early years are when the parents start to develop habits for their children, and the earlier they start, the better. With the increase in obesity consciousness in the United States and the increase in the awareness that obesity prevention begins in infancy, this task is becoming easier, at least with certain parents.

Inquire about the health habits of the parents. Ask about the intake of fruits, vegetables, grains, types of meats, and fast foods. Ask the parents if they exercise regularly and what plan they follow. The answers to these questions will give you an idea of the amount of regular exercise counseling that the family requires. The biggest challenge for clinicians, as well as the most important role for a clinician when prescribing regular exercise, is counseling families on how to implement the exercise prescription. This is the element that will have the biggest impact on future health for the child. The earlier healthy eating and regular exercise habits begin in the life of a child, the easier it is to maintain these habits as the child ages. Ensuring good eating habits at this young age is, in theory at least, very simple. The parent is the one supplying the food for the baby to eat. They need to make sure the foods are all healthy: fruits, vegetables, whole grains, lean meats, and legumes. This is very easy in the first two years of life, but it will be very helpful if the practice is reinforced at each visit.

The implementation of the exercise prescription itself can start at birth. Counsel both parents to exercise on a regular basis with their baby. Encourage parents to be physically active and to bring their baby with them when they exercise. The formation of exercise classes with babies is a new trend and one that clinicians should encourage. All children learn behavior by example, and the parent should be advised to model good exercise habits because ***their*** exercise behavior is the most important ingredient of the exercise prescription at this point in their child's development.

Activities that parents can do with their *toddlers* include taking them for walks, going to playgrounds, taking them swimming, or engaging in any physical play or game. All this will encourage a toddler to move around and be active. At the same time, it is important to reduce the amount of time that the television is used as a babysitter. Counsel the parents about the detrimental effects of too much television-watching. Increased television time is associated with increased risk for obesity, as well as the possibility of increased violent behavior. The attraction to child-oriented shows is very strong at this age, but the parent should be encouraged to be a strong parent and limit this sedentary activity (22).

The visits between 2–3 years should be the start of the dialogue between you and your patient. Children can understand language at this developmental stage and will have fun engaging the clinician in a conversation. Start to talk with the children about how they are eating and how strong they are. Children love to show off their muscles, and if the clinician encourages them to do so, they can use the opportunity to tell them how to keep strong. Parents should be instructed on the developmental capability of a 2–3 year old, and exercise counseled accordingly. Play time should be the main focus of this age group. Encourage running, jumping, squatting, as well as swimming with the parents. Throwing, catching, and squeezing balls are all excellent forms of activity for children of this age. It is very important to remind parents that all activity must be supervised by an adult at all times.

3–6-Year-Olds

Developmental abilities are changing rapidly in this age group. Children can pedal a bicycle. They can hop on one foot and skip. The social climate also changes drastically at this age. Pre-school brings friends and social groups and even team sports. For this age group, you can encourage 60 minutes of fun exercise activity on most days of the week. Scheduled classes offered at gyms, karate classes, and swimming classes should be encouraged. Along with "scheduled" exercise, team-sport activities like soccer and T-ball begin during this age group. If the child does not like team sports, then encourage the parent to investigate other physical activities, like tennis and swimming, for example. A home routine of regular exercise can easily be developed for this age group. You can use the exercise regimen in the book. Photocopy the pages and give them to your patients. Many of the exercises use resistance training with the child's body weight as the resistance.

6–12-Year-Olds

The elementary school years presents new developmental changes and challenges. Competitive sports begin and the social scene takes on a new life. The number of times the children are seen in the office decreases, so each encounter needs to be a forum to instill the regular exercise prescription. There will be a percentage of children who are participating in a team sport. Encourage the children to continue the sport, but also ask about how often the team meets for practice and games. Review the practice routine with the child. Since most organized sports concentrate more on learning and mastering the sport rather than teaching the children about the proper way to exercise, clinicians can fill this gap by continuing to counsel families to try to have their children exercise for 60 minutes on most days of the week and that pre- and post-exercise or team practice stretching is essential to regular exercise. The days that the children are engaged in team sports or exercise classes are counted toward the daily 60-minute exercise recommendation.

It is unlikely that a team practices more than three times a week in this age group; therefore, you should encourage other forms of regular exercise in order to reach the weekly regular exercise prescription. Encourage exercise that includes the entire family: bike riding, swimming, skiing, hiking, dancing, jogging, walking, and outdoor games like basketball and catch. The exercise requirement does not need to be done all at one time. The day can be broken up into a 15-minute calisthenics routine and a 45-minute walk after dinner, for example. The family can break up the exercise into any bits of time (that add up to 60 minutes) that works best for them. Reinforce resistance training as part of the program and give them a copy of the exercise program in this book.

The Teenage Years

For adolescents, motivational interviewing (see Chaps 4–6) is imperative to helping them start regular exercise or to keep them on a regular exercise routine. The motivational interview is very effective for this age group, because the focus is on the teenager's likes and desires. The clinician will focus on the positive aspects of exercise and how maintaining health will help them achieve their future goals. Use activities that the adolescent enjoys participating in to help them with an exercise program. Social issues are of the utmost importance in this age group and local exercise facilities can provide socialization and exercise at the same time.

Sunday	Monday	Tuesday	Wednesday	Thursday	Friday	Saturday
	Activity class	Home exercise	Activity class	Home exercise	Home exercise	Activity class or
	Team sport 45–60 Minutes	30 Minutes	Team sport 45–60 Minutes	30 Minutes	30 Minutes	team sport 45–60 Minutes
Indoor or outdoor fun play	Indoor or outdoor fun play	Indoor or outdoor fun play	Indoor or outdoor fun play	Indoor or outdoor fun play	Indoor or outdoor fun play	Indoor or outdoor fun play

Some exercise facilities allow adolescents to use the facility after the age of 13 years. If the patient is emotionally mature, encourage the patient to use a facility with supervision. An exercise routine should include 10 minutes of warming up and stretching to prepare the body for exercise and reduce injury. This should be followed by 30 minutes of a vigorous cardiac exercise and a warm-down for five minutes to bring the heart rate down. The exercise routine should end with 15–20 minutes of resistance training.

It is very important to talk with adolescents on the proper use of weights when exercising. They must avoid hyperextension of the spine and maximal lifts. A maximal lift is the maximum amount of weight that can be lifted with proper form for one repetition. Adolescent males are at risk for engaging in maximal lifts. Lifting a maximal amount of weight for one repetition can cause significant damage to bone, muscle, tendon, or ligaments. The greatest risk of physical damage occurs just before the onset of puberty. This information needs to be conveyed to every family. The amount of weight to be lifted should be weight that can be lifted for 10–15 repetitions while maintaining proper technique. The rest period between each set should be three times as long as the time it took to do one set of repetitions. Once the repetitions can be done without muscle fatigue, the weight can be increased by 5%–10%.

Team sports in this age group often require vigorous training on most days of the week and usually provide enough physical activity for the adolescent. The motivation for adolescents to participate in vigorous team sports is varied and usually is not based on preventing future health problems. This should not preclude the clinician from continuing to inform the patient about all the benefits that this activity is having for their health. For adolescents who don't like team sports, or don't qualify for them for one reason or another, regular exercise outside of them must be emphasized. Exercise must continue through summer and off-season. Statistics show that as adolescents move through high school, fewer and fewer of them participate in team sports. If they do not learn to maintain an exercise program without a team, the exercise habit can be lost (23).

If families who live in cities are unable to participate in outdoor activities, the indoor exercise program will work well. Another option is some of the new video exercise games or "exergames." Video games are one of the most popular forms of entertainment for children and the makers of them have come out with games that can burn calories while children play them. If the family owns a game system, encourage them to purchase video games that require physical interaction.

SAMPLE REGULAR EXERCISE PRESCRIPTION

Following is a sample home exercise program (7) that provides a cardiovascular and resistance workout with flexibility training for children three years and older. No equipment is required except a clock to keep time. Play some music and have fun.

Time	Exercise
	THE WARM-UP
1 Minute	Light jogging in place
1 Minute	Continue with jogging but add arm rolls
1 Minute	While still jogging in place, change to arm pull backs
	Slow down to a stop and while standing do a quadriceps stretch for a count of 10 on each leg
	Down on the floor and do a hamstring stretch for a count of 10 on each leg
	Back stretch. Sit on the floor with your legs straight out in front of you. Cross your left leg over the right leg and place your right arm around your left leg. Slowly turn your body toward the left while keeping your spine straight. Hold for a count of 10. Repeat on the other side.

EXERCISE TIME

20 Jumping Jacks

20 bicycle sit ups with head and shoulders off the floor

20 Jumping Jacks

10 squat thrusts

20 jumping jacks

10 push ups

20 jumping jacks

10 squats

20 jumping jacks

10 chin ups using a chin up bar

60 jumping jacks

THE WARM-DOWN

March in place for 1 minute to slow the heart rate down.

Forward bend and stretch for a count of 20.

Lie flat on the floor and do an overhead stretch.

Bend and roll your legs to the right. Keeping your shoulders on the mat and hold for a count of 20. Roll and repeat on the other side.

Sit up slowly and make a v with your legs. Lean forward stretching your inner thighs. Do not roll your spine. Picture a target between your legs about a foot high and try to reach for it. Hold for a count of 10.

Now reach to your left. Picture a target about 1 foot above your toes and try to reach for it. Hold for a count of 10. Repeat on the other side.

CONCLUSION

This chapter is about the important health benefits of prescribing regular exercise in the pediatric population, strategies on how to advise families in achieving their regular exercise goals, and assistance in counseling families on how to overcome the barriers to regular exercise. It is evident that in order for the exercise prescription to be successful, exercise must be a *regular, family affair,* and as much as possible about *fun* (24). As a parent models behavior for their children, you are in the unique position to be able to model behaviors for your patients and their families, if you choose to do so. By practicing regular exercise and by prescribing regular exercise at all visits, you can influence an entire family's future health and have a long-lasting impact for years to come.

References

1. *ACSM's Guidelines for Exercise Testing and Prescription*
2. Hebestreit HU, Bar-Or O. Differences between children and adults for exercise testing and prescription. In: Skinner JS, editor. Exercise testing and exercise prescription for special cases. Philadelphia (PA): Lippincott Williams & Wilkins; 2005. p. 68–84.
3. Roach RC, Stepanek J, Hackett PH. Acute mountain sickness and high-altitude cerebral edema. In: Lounsbury DE, Bellamy RF, Zajtchuk R, editors. Medical aspects of harsh environments. Washington: Office of the Surgeon General (US), Borden Institute; 2002. p. 765–93.
4. Olshansky SJ, et al. A Potential Decline in Life Expectancy in the United States in the 21st Century, NEJM, Volume 352, 1138–1145, March 2005.

CHAPTER 15

Finding the Fun in Regular Exercise

Steven Jonas

INTRODUCTION

To begin, what do we mean by "fun"? First, the activity itself can be fun, whether it's feeling good about climbing the stairs to the office every day, going out for a bike ride on a Sunday morning, getting out in the fresh air on a walk, or spending time at the gym doing exercises that are enjoyable in one way or another (and not doing the ones that are not). Second, adding "externals," as we detail below in "settings, surroundings, and companions," can be fun. Third, certain outcomes of becoming and being a regular exerciser, like travel that focuses on exercise (walking, cycling, and hiking tours) or exercising in different settings while traveling (which we discuss later in this chapter) can make exercise fun. Finally, for many regular exercisers the mental and physical outcomes they experience once they are into it are fun in and of themselves.

For many people who are thinking about regular exercise, "will it be fun?" or, conversely, "won't it be not fun?" are questions that early come to mind. Many people don't want to start because they are afraid that it just won't be fun, that it will be work. Some think: "This is going to be terrible. I'm going to hate it, every step of the way. But I've got to do it. I've got to get into shape." However, if it does not eventually become fun in one way or another, most people will not continue with it, whether it is through lifestyle exercise (LE) or leisure-time scheduled exercise (LTSE), or some combination of both.

It happens that for many people who start one program or another, even with a negative attitude, exercising at some level eventually turns out to be fun of one kind or another anyway. Sometimes even in just a few weeks, they find that they are enjoying themselves at the physical or mental level or both. However, if your patient can get started with a positive attitude, they will improve their chances of having fun, which of course improves their chances of staying with it and then having fun in one or more of the ways listed above and discussed further below. You can help by helping them to attend to one or more of the details discussed below. For your convenience in dealing with your patients on this subject, the voicing for the balance of this chapter is addressed directly to your patient.

MENTAL PREPARATION

If you can manage it, positive anticipation is a very important element in having fun while exercising regularly. It can be fun if you can find the way(s) *to let it be fun.*

That process begins with all of the mental preparation that is a principal focus of this book. First, of course, is carefully setting goals *for* the exercise that are appropriate for *you.* If at the outset they appear to be too tough, trying to get there won't be fun. Neither will it be if they are too easy. Second, as we have stressed repeatedly, it is essential to not do too much, too soon, whether in LE or LTSE. Third, it is essential to focus first on the regular, then on the exercise. Fourth is the importance of understanding that it is gradual change that leads to permanent changes. Fifth, it is recognizing the fact that for many, the exercise they choose can indeed become fun itself, as well as being fun for the results it will produce. (See Three-Minute Drill 15-1.)

For some, the most fun of the regular exercise experience happens when they learn how to *use their training sessions for thinking.* You can plan your day if you work out in the morning, or review your day if you work out in the evening. You can think about projects you are working on. Some regular exercisers have experienced some of their most creative moments when out on a workout (the only problem being to try to remember the inspiration so that you can write it down when you get home!). If you have particularly nice thoughts that you want to revel in (or possibly personal problems that you need to deal with) concerning spouse, "significant other," children, or parents, your exercise time will provide you with some privacy just to do that thinking. *No phone, no interruptions from family or co-workers; just you, alone with your thoughts.*

Finally, you can give yourself *rewards for performance* in terms of weeks of exercise, total time, distance, increased speed in LTSE (if that's for you), and the like. The rewards can be clothing, special experiences such as deferred travel or going to a show, or a new piece of equipment. Self-rewarding does take a spe-

THREE-MINUTE DRILL, 15 – 1

Making Exercise Fun: The Mental Aspects

1. Let it be fun.
2. Set appropriate goals.
3. Don't do too much, too soon.
4. First on the regular, then on the exercise.
5. Understand that gradual change leads to permanent changes.
6. Recognize that the exercise chosen can become fun itself.
7. Recognize that the results can be fun, if given time.
8. Use the training sessions for thinking, when the activity chosen permits.
9. Anticipate rewards for performance.

cial kind of discipline, because there is nothing to stop you from engaging in those behaviors, anyway. However, if you can exert the self-discipline and then get the self-reward after getting to a certain self-selected point either in LE or LTSE, the behaviors are not only good for their own sakes, but they will also help make exercising regularly fun.

SETTINGS, SURROUNDINGS, AND COMPANIONS

One way to have fun is to *set non-exercise-related goals for the exercise session itself,* like getting an errand or two done in the course of it. Perhaps you will pick up your newspaper or a container of milk and a loaf of bread while you are out. Perhaps you will go to the Post Office. Perhaps your car needs to be dropped off for servicing. You can drive to the service station, leave the car, and bike, run, or PaceWalk™ home. When the car is ready to be picked up, you can reverse the sequence. For those who live in areas where there are other regular exercisers with whom you can work out out-of-doors (walkers, runners, cyclists) or go to a gym, doing so is a very good way to meet new friends. Other than gyms, city parks offer good opportunities of this type.

Especially for the LTSE approach, *setting up your training program in minutes, not miles,* is very helpful (and LE sessions are most often defined in minutes, anyway). Doing so will help you avoid the stress that can be created by worrying about either speed or distance. If you become a cyclist or a runner or a PaceWalker, you can add fun to your program and keep it there by *learning and using different routes.* Variety helps maintain interest for many people. Different routes can also present different challenges. If you are a cyclist, you could develop a hilly ride, one that is mostly flat, and one longer, combination route. On the other hand, you may find one favorite course that you will do over and over again, with slight variations to accommodate the changes in workout times laid out by TSTEP.

Doing your training sessions with a companion is one of the best ways to deal with boredom. There is nothing like good conversation (or even not-so-good conversation) to make a workout just fly by. (Of course, you will be giving up

THREE-MINUTE DRILL, 15 – 2

Settings, Surroundings, and Companions

1. Set non-exercise–related goals.
2. Set LTSE training programs in minutes, not miles.
3. Learn and use different routes.
4. Exercise with a companion.
5. Listen to music, the news, talk radio, and/or audio courses.
6. Take care for safety.

that private time we spoke of in the previous section.) However, if it is going to work for you, there are several problems with this approach that you will have to solve. You have to find the right partner (or partners). You will need someone with whom you can establish a common schedule and who works out at about your pace. This person also has to be someone with whom you have a good deal in common and with whom you can have interesting conversations, on a regular basis. Probably the most realistic approach is to find someone with whom you will be happy and comfortable working out with on occasion. You might also look for a walking, running, or cycling club in your area.

Some people find that *a companion of the canine variety* is ideal. Any conversation that you might have with your dog will be of the one-way variety. You don't have to talk when you don't feel like it. In most cases, your dog won't notice when you are ignoring him or her. Furthermore, you will always have the choice of topics of conversation. You don't have to discuss subjects that you don't like or make you feel uncomfortable. Dogs generally have as much stamina as you do, if not more, although that does vary by breed.

Ken McAlpine reviewed a listing of the running abilities of various breeds of dog which appeared in (believe it or not) a whole book devoted to the subject of running with one's dog (1). While a bulldog can manage only about 15 miles per week, Beagles, Cocker Spaniels, Great Danes, and St. Bernards can do about 25 miles per week; and Dalmatians, English setters, German shepherds, Golden Retrievers, and Siberian Huskies can handle about 35 miles per week. Most dogs other than the really large-sized ones like the Danes and the St. Bernards, can begin running regularly when they reach about one year of age. Of course you do have to train dogs to understand that regularly exercising and dog walking are two different things. Your dog has to know that stops at fire-hydrants and lamp-posts, to get acquainted with other dogs, and to sniff out the most interesting odors in the neighborhood are appropriate for the latter, not the former. Once this training is accomplished, your dog will generally trot along, right at your pace.

Finally, you can establish an internal setting to make regular exercise fun by *listening to music, the news, talk radio, and/or audio courses* while you work out. Also, there are audio tapes with rhythmic music played at various cadences, useful in PaceWalking™ or running. There is a wide variety of radios, tape and CD players, as well as the I-pod and similar devices that you can use while running, PaceWalking™, indoor cycling and rowing, stair-climbing, and the like. A head-set can make an LE session that consists of getting off rapid transit a stop or two before your destination more fun too.

There are safety considerations. Carrying a radio/cassette player in your hand while working out is not a good idea. It can easily lead to muscular imbalance, pain, and even injury. You should strap it around your arm or place it in a belt-carrier. When you are exercising out-of-doors, you must be able to hear as well as see potential danger. Thus, for music/radio listeners, there are three notes of caution to bear in mind, all in the interest of safety. First, you must have your ear channels open to the outside world so that you can hear impending dangers, such as an automobile rapidly approaching from behind you. Never use a headset where the speakers are designed to plug fully into the ear. Use only the "air-flow" type with the little sponge, or the mini-speakers that either stand perpendicularly to the side of your head or balance over the entrance to the ear canal without blocking it.

Second, of course, don't play the music too loudly. That's not safe, and you could also damage your hearing. Third, never listen to a portable stereo while cycling on the road. Of all regular exercisers, cyclists are the most prone to injury from external causes: motor vehicles, people, animals, other cyclists, road conditions. For safety, you must concentrate fully on the road or trail. If you find cycling boring without the benefit of such a distraction, it is better to pick another sport than to try to solve the problem by listening to music while cycling.

OF PLACE AND TIME

If your LE or LTSE approach takes you outdoors, you may find that you *appreciate the changing of the seasons* in a way you never did before. In the winter, when properly dressed, a run or a PaceWalk on a sunny, cold, crisp day can be marvelously invigorating. The summertime is great for those who like working up a hefty sweat. If you are properly dressed (this time on the light side), don't try to go too fast, and make sure that you get enough water to drink; those training sessions can be invigorating too. The best times of year for most people, however, are the spring and the fall, when the sun is shining and the temperature is just right. Virtually any exercise done then really connects you with the great outdoors.

Speaking of seasonal variation, observing it up close and personal can add an element of fun for the outdoors regular exerciser. From the new greenery appearing each spring, through the changing of the leaves in the fall, and the crispness of the snow in the winter (do wear the right shoes and watch where you are going, though!), observing the signs of the changing seasons can add a fun element to outdoor exercising.

Exercising while traveling can be fun, too. If work or tourism takes you away from home, you will have opportunities to add spice to your exercise program. If you travel to different cities on business, try to plan some time for at least one training session in each one. Just a few of the fun venues around the United States are:

- Central Park in New York City's borough of Manhattan. There is a reservoir located in the northern half of the park. Circling it is a 1.6 mile cinder path, a protected place to run or PaceWalk. The Park drives provide varied routes up to 6 plus miles in length. They are open to vehicular traffic only during weekday rush hours, and even then one lane is reserved for pedestrians and cyclists. In New York City also there is a running/walking/cycling path along the Hudson River from mid-town down to the Battery, and north of it, Riverside Park offers similar routes up to 116th street.

- Chicago's Lake Front, in sight of the famous sky-line, offers several miles of flat pedestrian paths for running or walking.
- In Fort Worth, Texas, the Trinity Trail, open to walkers, runners, and cyclists, runs for miles along the banks of the Trinity River. It is a quiet, smooth path, with no vehicular traffic.
- The Federal area of Washington, D.C., offers many miles of flat paths with views of the Potomac River, our national monuments, and elegant government buildings. A short distance away, there is some gentle hill running in Rock Creek Park.
- Brooklyn, New York's Prospect Park has a lovely 3.4-mile park drive loop reserved for walkers, runners, and cyclists during most daylight hours of the week.
- There are miles of protected pathways for walkers, runners, and cyclists along the banks of Charles River that separates Boston and Cambridge, MA. And the views are magnificent.
- In Philadelphia, PA, The Parkway, a broad boulevard, leads from the business district to the Fine Arts Museum. There you can go up the steps with the "Rocky" theme playing in your head and stop at the site of the statue of Philadelphia's most famous fictional character. For a change of pace, you can then proceed along a winding, tree-lined path bordering the Schuylkill River for several miles.
- In San Francisco, CA, running or walking up and down the various routes over Nob Hill is a breathtaking experience (in more ways than one). If you like your running/walking flat, with views too, try the Embarcadero.
- New Orleans, LA, offers riverside running or walking both on restored river park pathways, and on the roads the old wharf section, alongside the mighty Mississippi.
- In San Diego, CA, try the Old Town, where local walking clubs happen to be very active.
- There is not too much comfortable running in Los Angeles, CA, because of the smog, but if you like hill running or walking and can get over to Beverly Hills, try it. You will find the community to have been aptly named.
- In Boston, MA, with the completion of the "Big Dig," you can comfortably walk and run alongside the old Boston Harbor.

It happens that with a little perseverance you can discover in most cities in the United States (and many cities abroad for that matter) fine, stimulating places to exercise. As a general rule, waterfronts/riverfronts often provide excellent running/walking opportunities.

ENJOYING THE SPORTS FOR THEIR OWN SAKE

Many of the sports from among which you can choose for the LTSE approach are naturally rhythmic: PaceWalking™, running, cycling, swimming, aerobic dance, rowing. You may well find this aspect of your sport enjoyable for its own sake. You can really get into that smoothness, that flow, that feeling of being in control of your body, making it do things that it hasn't done before. You move rhythmically and you breath rhythmically. Many of the things we do in life have no rhythm; exercise does.

As we have noted, if you have the skill and the interest, you can work out doing the appropriate competitive sports. The racquet and team sports are of course inherently fun. If you are doing them primarily as part of an aerobic exercise program, you of course have to make sure that you are doing them aerobically. In tennis, for example, that means that you have to be a reasonably skilled player, you have to play against people who are at least as good as you are, and you have to play singles with a good deal of running. It is easier to maintain an aerobic level in squash or racquet ball than it is in tennis, as long as neither of you spends a lot of time standing around at change of service. In basketball, you must play full-court and in a game where fouls result in taking the ball out-of-bounds, not taking foul-shots.

Of course, if you are not worried about whether the exercise is aerobic, then these sports are fine whether you do them aerobically or not. The major disadvantages of these kinds of sports for your program is that they require one or more other people to do them with, court space which usually has to be reserved in advance, and a regular schedule. Again, you might think about a competitive sport as one component of a multisport program, which brings us to Pace-Training (see also Chapter 11, pp. 168–180). Pace-Training, setting up a program in which you do more than one sport/athletic activity, is one of the best ways to make regular exercise fun. This approach to exercising regularly adds variety and reduces the risk of overuse injury related to any one of the sports you include in it, as compared with doing just one of them exclusively.

Finally, if you are engaging in one or more of the distance sports, doing a race now and again can add a great deal of fun to your program (see also Chapter 11). In most parts of the country, you can readily find running races to do, and if you are a PaceWalker, you can always walk rather than run the course of a running road race if you so choose. In any case, regardless of the gait you use, you don't have to worry about speed. You will find that at least three-quarters of the entrants in any road race are out there just to have a good time. They are concerned with neither speed nor winning, but rather with crossing the finish line happily and healthily. If you are concerned about finishing last, rest assured that in any race there is almost always at least one person who is slower than you are. In any case, it's better to finish last than, say, sixth from last. When you are last, everyone knows who you are: when sixth from last, you are completely anonymous.

There are two principal reasons why you might want to try racing. First, races are just plain fun. You engage in your sport (or in the case of triathlon/duathlon, sports) with some drive to push yourself a bit in terms of speed and/or distance on that particular day. You can get to meet many healthy, nice, interesting people, most of whom, like you, are there simply to participate and complete the course. Only a very few have any potential for winning, either overall or in their age class. Thus, there is very little competitiveness. There is just a big group of people out to have a good time, going as fast as they can or feel like going on that particular day.

Second, racing can help to deal with potential boredom in an LTSE program. Racing can provide a good focus for your training. If you race, you have something specific to train for. You have a series of events on your calendar which break up the training year or season into manageable pieces. You create for yourself a set of peaks around which you can drape your training schedule. Finally, racing itself can keep you going as a regular exerciser where you might otherwise not do it or might do it for considerably less time and with considerably less intensity.

You can locate races through, for example, national and local running, cycling, swimming, and triathlon publications and Web sites, and at local "pro-shop" running shoe and bicycle stores.

BUILDING IN VARIETY AND TAKING TIME OFF

Building variety into your program, whether you are using the lifestyle exercise, or the leisure-time scheduled exercise approach, or some combination of both, is very helpful for making regular exercise fun on a year-round basis. Further, once you have become a regular exerciser and know that you are going to continue being one, as previously noted, we highly recommend that you take some time off, for a week or two, 1–2 times/year. Doing so gives both your body and your mind some needed rest and will be very helpful in keeping you going over time. You will not lose very much of your conditioning, if any, by resting for that short a period of time every now and then. You may be surprised to discover that once you have established regular exercise as a regular part of your life, it may be difficult to stand down. You may be finding yourself missing "your exercise fix," but stand down, anyway. It's good for you over the long run. We, the authors, can only hope that what we have had to share with you and your clinicians in this book will help you to reach the point that you will indeed feel that way about regular exercise.

And so, as we noted at the beginning of this chapter: regular exercise can be fun if you let it be fun.

Reference

1. McAlpine K. Canines compared. Runner's World. 1993 Apr:19. Citing Running with man's best friend. Crawford (CO): Alpine Publications; 1986.

GLOSSARY

AACVPR—American Association of Cardiovascular and Pulmonary Rehabilitation

ACOG—American College of Obstetrics and Gynecology

ACSM—American College of Sports Medicine

BMD—Bone mineral density

CABG—Coronary artery bypass graft surgery

CAD—Coronary artery disease

CDC—Centers for Disease Control and Prevention

CHF—Congestive heart failure

Chronometer—digital stopwatch

CPR—Cardio-pulmonary resuscitation

CPT—Certified Personal Trainer^{SM}

CVD—Cardiovascular disease

DASH—Dietary Approaches to Stop Hypertension

DBP—Diastolic blood pressure

DOMS—Delayed Onset Muscle Soreness

ECG—Electrocardiogram

ES—Exercise Specialist®

FAST—Foundation Aerobic SporT

FITT—Frequency, Intensity, Time (or duration), and Type

Five As Framework: Assess, Advise, Agree, Assist, Arrange follow-up

GDM—Gestational diabetes mellitus

GPS—Global positioning system

GXT—Graded exercise test

HDL-C—High-density lipoprotein cholesterol

HFI—Health/Fitness Instructor®

HR$_{max}$—Maximal heart rate

HRR—Heart rate reserve

ICD—Implantable cardioverter defibrillator

KSAs—Knowledge, Skills, and Attitudes

LE—Lifestyle exercise

LTSE—Leisure-time scheduled exercise

LDL-C—Low-density lipoprotein cholesterol

MDD—Major depressive disorder

METs—Metabolic equivalents

NIH—National Institutes of Health

PaceTraining—Working out in two or more sports on a regular basis in the same program, for health, fitness, and fun

PaceWalking™—"Exercise walking," "power walking," "fitness walking;" walking fast using a defined technique that differs from that of ordinary walking

PAD—Peripheral arterial disease

PAR-Q—Physical Activity Readiness Questionnaire

PTCA—Percutaneous transluminal coronary angioplasty

RCEP—Registered Clinical Exercise Physiologist®

RMR—Resting metabolic rate

RPE—Rating of Perceived Exertion

SBP—Systolic blood pressure

Six Stages of Change—Precontemplation, contemplation, preparation, action, maintenance, and termination.

SMART—Specific, Measurable, Achievable, Realistic, and Time-Bound

Three Ms—Mentioning, Motivating, Modeling

THR—Target heart rate

TSTEP—The Scheduled Training Exercise Program

USPSTF—U.S. Preventive Services Task Force

VO$_{2max}$—Maximal oxygen consumption

VO$_2$R—Oxygen consumption reserve

WMP—Wellness Motivational Pathway

RESOURCES

Active Living Every Day
Human Kinetics/Active Living Partners
1607 North Market Street
P.O. Box 5076
Champaign, IL 61825-5076
Phone: 217-351-5076
Fax: 217-351-2674
http://www.activeliving.info/

Activity Calorie Calculator
http://www.primusweb.com/fitnesspartner/
jumpsite/calculat.htm

Aerobics and Fitness Association
of America
15250 Ventura Blvd., Suite 200
Sherman Oaks, CA 91403
Phone: 1-877-YOUR-BODY
(1-877-968-7263)
http://www.afaa.com/

American Academy of Podiatric
Sports Medicine
Phone: 888-854-FEET
http://www.aapsm.org/index.html

American Alliance for Health, Physical
Education, Recreation & Dance
1900 Association Drive
Reston, VA 20191
1-800-213-7193
info@aahperd.org
http://www.aahperd.org/

American Association of Cardiovascular
and Pulmonary Rehabilitation
401 North Michigan Avenue, Suite 2200
Chicago, IL 60611
Phone: 312-321-5146
Fax: 312-673-6924
http://www.aacvpr.org/

American College of Obstetrics
and Gynecology
409 12th St., S.W.
PO Box 96920
Washington, DC 20090-6920
Phone: 202-638-5577
www.acog.org

American College of Preventive Medicine
1307 New York Avenue, N.W., Suite 200
Washington, DC 20005
Tel: (202) 466-2044
Fax: (202) 466-2662
Email: info@acpm.org
www.acpm.org

American College of Sports Medicine
401 West Michigan Street
Indianapolis, IN 46202-3233
Phone: 317-637-9200
Fax: 317-634-7817
http://www.acsm.org

(ACE) American Council on Exercise
4851 Paramount Drive
San Diego, CA 92123
Phone: 1-858-279-8227
Phone: 1-888-825-3636
Fax: (858) 279-8064
http://www.acefitness.org/

American Heart Association National Center
7272 Greenville Avenue
Dallas, TX 75231
AHA: 1-800-AHA-USA-1 or 1-800-242-8721
ASA: 1-888-4-STROKE or 1-888-478-7653
AHA Professional Membership: 1-800-787-
8984 or Outside US: 1-301-223-2307
AHA Instructor Network:
1-877-AHA-4CPR
http://www.americanheart.org

255

American Physical Therapy Association
1111 North Fairfax Street
Alexandria, VA 22314-1488
800/999-APTA (2782)
703/684-APTA (2782)
TDD: 703/683-6748
Fax: 703/684-7343
http://www.apta.org//AM/Template.cfm?
Section=Home

Apollo Hospitals
www.ewellnessrx.com

Centers for Disease Control and Prevention
1600 Clifton Rd
Atlanta, GA 30333
Phone: 404-498-1515 or 800-311-3435
Growing stronger—Strength training for older adults
http://www.cdc.gov/nccdphp/dnpa/physical
/growing_stronger/why.htm.

IDEA Health & Fitness Association
10455 Pacific Center Court
San Diego, CA 92121-4339
Phone: 800.999.4332, ext. 7
Fax: 858.535.8234
http://www.ideafit.com

Institute of Lifestyle Medicine
Department of Physical Medicine and
Rehabilitation, Harvard Medical School
Spaulding Rehabilitation Hospital
125 Nashua Street
Boston, MA 02114
Phone: 508 532 4241
http://www.instituteoflifestylemedicine.org

Institute for Aerobics Research
The Cooper Institute
12330 Preston Road
Dallas, TX 75230
Phone: 972-341-3200
Fax: 972-341-3227
Toll-Free (USA): 800-635-7050
http://www.cooperinst.org/index.cfm

International Dance-Exercise Association
10455 Pacific Center Court
San Diego, CA 92121-4339
Phone: 800-999-4332, ext. 7
Fax: 858-535-8234
http://www.ideafit.com/

Jewish Community Center
520 Eighth Avenue
New York, NY 10018
Phone: 212-532-4949
Fax: 212-481-4174
http://www.jcca.org/

Kaiser Permanente
http://www.kaiserpermanente.org/

Mayo Clinic
Weight training exercises for major
muscle groups
http://www.mayoclinic.com/health/
weight-training/SM00041&slide=2

Medical Fitness Association
P.O. Box 73103
Richmond, VA 23235-8026
Call us: 804-897-5701
Fax us: 804-897-5704
http://www.medicalfitness.org

National Athletic Trainers' Association
2952 Stemmons Freeway Dallas, TX 75247
Phone: 214-637-6282
Fax: 214-637-2206
http://www.nata.org

**National Coalition for Promoting
Physical Activity**
1100 H Street, NW, Suite 510
Washington, DC 20005
http://www.ncppa.org/

**National Institutes of Health Senior Health
Web site**
Exercise for older adults.
Exercises to try—balance exercises.
http://nihseniorhealth.gov/exercise/
balanceexercises/01.html

National Strength and Conditioning Association
1885 Bob Johnson Drive
Colorado Springs, CO 80906
Phone: 719-632-6722
Fax: 719-632-6367
Toll-Free: 800-815-6826
http://www.nsca-lift.org/

PACE Project
Patient-Centered Assessment and
Counseling for Exercise and Nutrition
http://www.paceproject.org/Home.html

PAR-Q
Canadian Society for Exercise Physiology
185 Somerset St. West, Suite 202
Ottawa, Ontario CANADA K2P 0J2
Tel.: (613) 234-3755
Fax: (613) 234-3565
Toll-Free: 1-877-651-3755
http://www.csep.ca

President's Council on Physical Fitness and Sport
Department W
200 Independence Ave., SW
Room 738-H
Washington, DC 20201-0004
Phone: 202-690-9000
Fax: 202-690-5211
http://www.fitness.gov/

Tri-Hard Sports Conditioning
c/o Jason Gootman
22 Tracy Lyn Road
Holliston, MA 01746
508.429.5375
http://www.tri-hard.com/

U.S. Department of Health & Human Services
200 Independence Avenue, S.W.
Washington, DC 20201
202-619-0257
Toll Free: 1-877-696-6775
http://www.hhs.gov/

U.S. Preventive Services Task Force
Agency for Healthcare Research
and Quality
540 Gaither Road Rockville, MD 20850
Phone: 301-427-1364
http://www.ahrq.gov/clinic/USpstfix.htm

United States Public Health Service's Office of Disease Prevention and Health Promotion
1101 Wootton Parkway, Suite LL100
Rockville, MD 20852
Phone: 240-453-8280
Fax: 240-453-8282
http://odphp.osophs.dhhs.gov/

Wellcoaches Corporation
19 Weston Rd
Wellesley, MA, USA 02482
Toll Free: 1-866-WE-COACH or
866.932.6224 x702
http://www.wellcoach.com

YMCA of the USA
101 North Wacker Drive
Chicago, IL 60606
(800) 872-9622
http://www.ymca.net/

INDEX

Page numbers in *italics* denote figures; page numbers followed by *t* indicate tables.